PAIN-FREE WITH CBD

PAIN-FREE
WITH
CBD

EVERYTHING YOU NEED TO KNOW
to SAFELY and EFFECTIVELY
USE CANNABIDIOL

ALICE O'LEARY RANDALL
and ELOISE THEISEN

**ROCKRIDGE
PRESS**

Interior and Cover Designer: Linda Snorina
Art Producer: Hillary Frileck
Editors: Stacy Wagner-Kinnear and Vanessa Ta
Production Editor: Kurt Shulenberger

Copyright page credit: Shutterstock/prizma, p. 10; Shutterstock/Creativan, p. 32; Shutterstock/Irina Imago, p. 33; Shutterstock/AppleZoomZoom, p. 33; Shutterstock/Eskymaks, p. 34; Shutterstock/CAPJAH, p. 34; Shutterstock/ADragan, p. 38; Shutterstock/Enriscapes, p. 38; Creative Market/WebAndCat, p. 39.

Author Photo: Alice O'Leary Randall author photo courtesy of ©Marty Sterling Eubank

ISBN: Print 978-1-64152-554-1 | eBook 978-1-64152-555-8

R0

To Robert C. Randall
How could we ever have imagined?

CONTENTS

INTRODUCTION

Imagine prohibiting a substance with a 5,000-year history of use as a medicine, and then imagine restricting research on that drug to determine if there were indeed medical uses. You have just imagined the modern history of cannabis, better known as marijuana.

For more than three-quarters of a century, beginning in 1937, there has been a near global prohibition of cannabis. This prohibition effectively inhibited research with the drug but did little to stop its social use. In the late 1960s, I was in college and used marijuana recreationally, as did my husband, Robert C. Randall. In the early 1970s, Robert, then 24, was told he had glaucoma and would be blind by the time he was 30, but he accidentally discovered that smoking marijuana helped lower his eye pressures. We were arrested in 1975 for growing marijuana, but we fought the charges and won based on the defense of medical necessity. In 1976, Robert gained legal access to federal supplies of marijuana to treat his glaucoma, and news of his case led to the medical marijuana movement, of which my late husband is the acknowledged founder.

It is 43 years later and medical marijuana—more correctly, medical cannabis—is now well known around the world. Dozens of states and countries have enacted laws allowing the medicinal use of cannabis. For decades the focus has been on delta-9 tetrahydrocannabinol (THC), the component in cannabis that causes the commonly associated "high." That began to change in the early 21st century when another component of cannabis—cannabidiol, or CBD—began to claim the spotlight.

CBD exploded into global consciousness in 2013 when CNN produced the documentary *Weed*. Dr. Sanjay Gupta, the producer, who was also once staunchly against medical cannabis, told the world about a young girl, Charlotte Figi, with intractable epilepsy and how cannabis, in particular its component CBD, helped her control her seizures. There was even a CBD tincture named after her: Charlotte's Web.

Gupta also introduced his viewers to the endocannabinoid system (ECS), a unique physiological system that is present in all mammals. The ECS, discovered in the early 1990s, produces natural cannabinoids that link with cannabinoid receptors in every major organ of the body. When the body cannot produce enough natural cannabinoids, then cannabis becomes a substitute and a medicine. This discovery allowed scientists and researchers to begin understanding why cannabis is so helpful with such a wide spectrum of ailments. Research into cannabis, still tightly restricted in the United States, accelerated rapidly around the world, most particularly in Israel.

In 2014, the year after the first airing of the CNN documentary, I joined the board of directors of the American Cannabis Nurses Association (ACNA), and it was here that my education in CBD really began. Between 2014 and 2016 there were close to 20 states that adopted the so-called "CBD-only" laws. The intent behind these laws was to help children like Charlotte Figi, but as news and knowledge of CBD spread, there were more adults using CBD for a wide variety of ailments.

I, along with my ACNA colleagues, grew amazed at the rapid change in society's attitudes toward this "new" cannabis component. Some ACNA nurses began to talk about setting up cannabis-specific medical practices in states that had legal medical cannabis. Among them was Eloise Theisen, coauthor of chapter 3 of this book and a board-certified adult geriatric nurse pra-ctitioner from Northern California who had worked as an oncology nurse at John Muir Health.

Eloise saw the need for a cannabis-based medical practice that gave patients the opportunity to meet with a skilled healthcare practitioner, someone who would take the time to listen to and work with patients to find the right balance of cannabis medicine. In late 2014, with Dr. David Ferrera, Eloise established Green Health Consultants (now Radicle Health), possibly the first medical practice of its kind in the United States. In the years since, she has treated more than 5,000 patients using medical cannabis and CBD. I asked Eloise to assist me with chapter 3 in this book because of her hands-on experience with applying cannabis and CBD to real-time patients.

It's true that CBD does not work for everyone, but the odds are good it could help you. It behooves you to learn as much as you possibly can in order to use CBD efficiently. Our hope is this book will help you find the right solution to relieve *your* pain.

Alice O'Leary Randall

PART I
NATURE'S MEDICINE

CHAPTER ONE

HEALING WITHOUT A HIGH

CBD. You've seen the TV reports, read about it in the news, perhaps seen it on store shelves, or heard your friends sing its praises. You may have even heard it is good for your pet. There are claims that CBD helps with pain, digestive upset, insomnia, epilepsy, tremors, skin conditions, and more. Can anything be *this* good?

Yes! The therapeutic properties of CBD—its full name is cannabidiol—are numerous, diverse, and now being confirmed by modern research. Best of all, CBD may be able to replace some conventional medications that carry significant risks and numerous side effects. In particular, CBD has been shown effective in managing pain, and this book will show you how.

A Nation in Pain

Do you live with chronic pain? If so, you are not alone. There are 100 million Americans who live with chronic pain, and for many, finding relief from that pain has been an impossible task.

Chronic pain is described as pain lasting more than 12 weeks, and it can be brought on by many factors including disease, accident, or old age. The range of pain is extremely broad, from minor daily pain attributable to chronic ailments such as arthritis to debilitating pain that renders an individual incapable of functioning.

Remedies seem to abound, from over-the-counter pain relievers to strong narcotics. Pharmaceutical companies are constantly developing new drugs for pain relief, a situation that sadly led to an opioid crisis in the United States, which is still raging. In 2018, 68,000 people died from drug overdoses.[1] This crisis has led Americans to distrust pharmaceutical medicines. A Gallup poll conducted in 2017 found that 78 percent of Americans prefer to try other ways to treat physical pain before they take prescribed medication.[2] Other polls have demonstrated a growing interest in and use of natural or herbal supplements to maintain health.[3]

It is against this backdrop that CBD—cannabidiol—has exploded onto the scene as an alternative medicine for chronic pain.

Can CBD Help Me?

The answer to that question cannot be known for certain, but there are reasons to believe the answer is yes. CBD is just one component of the cannabis plant, which has a 5,000-year history of medical use,[4] in particular for pain. Scientists and entrepreneurs have developed ways to extract CBD from cannabis and hemp. It can be used safely, without concerns about the intoxicating side effects that are associated with CBD's molecular cannabis cousin, THC. This has led to a phenomenal situation in which people are now using CBD for a multitude of ailments. Search the web and you will find hundreds of anecdotal accounts of successful CBD use. Better yet, scientists are intrigued with this "new" medicine, and research is accelerating at a fantastic clip, with hundreds of scientific articles on CBD published every month.

Just a few of the ailments being successfully treated with CBD include inflammatory bowel disease, arthritis, lupus, ALS, anxiety, Parkinson's disease, multiple sclerosis, and more. CBD does not cure these ailments, but it can provide significant relief from associated pain and other symptoms.

CBD'S MEDICINAL PROPERTIES

Why is CBD so useful? Because it has an amazing number of properties that are helpful in the treatment of a multitude of ailments:

Anti-inflammatory: CBD helps reduce the pain of arthritis and other ailments.

Antianxiety: The calming properties of CBD make it appropriate for many illnesses.

Anticonvulsant: CBD helps people with epilepsy and traumatic brain injuries.

Neuroprotectant: Recovery and regeneration of the body's nervous system makes CBD especially useful for neuropathic peripheral pain and conditions such as Parkinson's disease and multiple sclerosis.

Strengthens immune system: A healthy immune system is obviously desirable, but many diseases, such as HIV and cancer, attack the immune system directly. CBD helps protect and restore the immune system.

Relieves pain: The combination of CBD's anti-inflammatory and neuroprotectant properties makes it an effective pain medication for many.

A CBD Glossary

Part of learning about CBD is understanding the language of cannabis. Here are a few important terms.

cannabis: This ancient herb is part of the *Cannabaceae* family. Varieties of cannabis include sativa, indica, and hemp.

CB1 and CB2 receptors: These receptors in the human body receive cannabinoids like CBD. The CB1 receptors are mainly in the brain (the central nervous system, or "CNS") but also in the lungs, liver, and kidneys. The CB2 receptors are mainly in the immune system and in hematopoietic blood production cells.

CBD: This is an abbreviation for cannabidiol, one of the principal cannabinoids of the cannabis plant.

ECS: This is an abbreviation for the endogenous cannabinoid system, a group of cannabinoid receptors located in the brain and throughout the human body. The ECS was discovered in the early 1990s; it is now known that the ECS is involved in a large number of physiological processes that help the human body stay balanced.

hemp: This variety of the cannabis sativa plant species is grown primarily for the industrial uses of its derived products. Hemp normally has less than 0.3 percent THC but does have CBD.

homeostasis: This describes the tendency of the human body to maintain internal stability. Homeostasis involves a coordinated response of the body to any situation or stimulus that would tend to disturb the body's balance.

marijuana: This is a slang term for cannabis.

neuroprotective: This means serving to protect nerve cells against damage, degeneration, or impairment of function. Various cannabinoids exhibit neuroprotective properties.

phytocannabinoids: These cannabinoids occur naturally in the cannabis plant ("phyto"). Endocannabinoids occur naturally in ("endo") the human body.

psychoactive: Any chemical substance that changes brain function and results in alterations in perception, mood, consciousness, or behavior is considered psychoactive.

THC: This is an abbreviation for tetrahydrocannabinol, one of at least 113 cannabinoids identified in cannabis. Delta-9 THC is the primary psychoactive consitutent of cannabis.

tincture: This liquid solution is typically an alcoholic extract of plant material. Numerous cannabinoid tinctures are available, including many CBD tinctures made from hemp.

Reduces side effects of cancer chemotherapy: CBD helps quell the nausea and vomiting associated with many chemotherapy drugs. And the anti-inflammatory and antianxiety properties can contribute to the patient's sense of well-being.

Calms the digestive tract: Our intestines have a multitude of receptors that are designed to receive CBD and promote healing.

Helps reduce substance abuse: Whether it is alcohol or drugs, CBD can help reduce the symptoms of withdrawal and help break the cycle of addiction.

What Is CBD?

In its simplest terms, CBD—cannabidiol—is a naturally occurring compound found in the cannabis plant. It is one of more than 100 cannabis compounds, called cannabinoids. These naturally occurring compounds are phytocannabinoids, meaning they occur in plants (*phyt-* is from the Greek and means plant). CBD is the most abundant compound in the cannabis plant. It is nonaddictive and nonintoxicating. But CBD is powerful. It can alter moods, affect the immune system, and even destroy cancer cells. What it does not do is get users high or intoxicated. THC, another cannabis compound, causes people to get high. Let's look at the difference between the two.

CBD IS NOT POT

Some people will say, "CBD is just like pot, only it doesn't get you high." Let's unpack that statement. First, pot is a slang term, one of more than 1,000 that exist for the cannabis plant. Cannabis is the proper scientific term for pot or marijuana, which is another slang term that arrived in the United States with Mexican immigrants in the early 20th century.

It is important to learn the proper terms and avoid slang when using cannabis or its compounds for medical purposes. High is another slang term that can be very misleading. It leads to statements like "CBD is nonpsychoactive," which is not entirely true. Many people equate psychoactive with intoxication, but, in its strictest form, psychoactive means "affecting the mind or behavior."[5] This is true for medications of all types, and CBD is no exception.

CANNABIS-DERIVED CBD

We have learned that CBD is a compound that originates from the cannabis plant, but as you start to learn more about CBD, you are going to see the following: "CBD derived from cannabis" and "CBD derived from hemp." What does that mean, and what's the difference?

First, let's establish that we are talking about natural CBD here. In both cases natural CBD is extracted from a plant: cannabis or hemp. While each of these plants is in the same phyto-family, the *Cannabaceae* family, within that plant family are several different species; the best known are cannabis indica and cannabis sativa. Throughout the ages, a subspecies of cannabis sativa developed, and it is called hemp. We will discuss hemp more in a bit.

Regardless of the cannabis variant, each contains over 100 compounds, including CBD and THC, but at varying proportions. The proportions and intensity of these compounds can be altered by farmers and scientists through various growing and laboratory methods.

HEMP-DERIVED CBD

Another misconception is that CBD from hemp is different from CBD derived from the cannabis plant. This is not accurate. There are, however, differences between cannabis and hemp. Most importantly, hemp has far less THC than regular cannabis plants. In fact, by law hemp plants must have less than 0.3 percent THC.[6]

Hemp is mainly an industrial plant, and recorded history is replete with mentions of the importance of hemp in the development of the civilized world. Well into the 20th century, hemp was used for paper, cloth, rope, textiles, shoes, insulation, biofuel, and even birdseed. But the Marijuana Tax Act of 1937 effectively eliminated hemp as well as cannabis.

Accessing Hemp-Derived CBD vs. Cannabis-Derived CBD

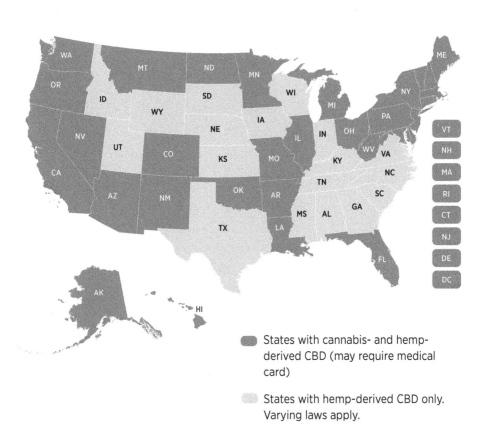

States with cannabis- and hemp-derived CBD (may require medical card)

States with hemp-derived CBD only. Varying laws apply.

When CBD began to emerge as an effective medical compound, hemp farmers began to realize this could be a new market for them. However, in addition to low THC content, traditional hemp also had a low content of CBD. As a result, great volumes of hemp were required in order to extract a worthy amount of CBD. This soon resulted in farmers and scientists working to modify hemp plants so as to permit the manufacture of greater amounts of CBD. Today, there are hemp variants that have both a very high proportion of CBD and a very low proportion of THC.

The Stigma of Cannabis

The growth and use of CBD have been made more complex by the stigma of cannabis and by the manner in which our society has dealt with it during recent years. More than 30 US states have legalized cannabis for medical purposes, but it remains against the federal law to use cannabis for medical purposes. If that is not confusing, then what is?

This confusion is the result of a misplaced, decades-long prohibition of cannabis. A great deal of false information was manufactured, not to control a dangerous drug but rather to control certain populations that were deemed "dangerous."

CANNABIS BEFORE THE 20TH CENTURY

The relationship of cannabis and mankind can be traced back literally thousands of years. Archaeologists have discovered ancient tombs with remnants of cannabis carefully laid next to the deceased. Early medical uses of cannabis can be traced to Chinese and Egyptian cultures that date back 5,000 years.[7]

Hemp has an equally long association with mankind. Some of the earliest recorded history is on paper made from hemp. The sailing ships of old had many hemp products on board, including rope and sails. Hemp clothing dates back 10,000 years, and archaeologists have found hemp cloth in Iraq that carbon dated to 8,000 years ago.[8]

Introduction of cannabis to Western medicine happened in the mid-1800s when Dr. William O'Shaugnessy returned to England from India, where he saw locals using cannabis, which they called ganja, to treat various ailments. In a time when most medicines were made from plants, cannabis was rapidly accepted. It was used to treat headaches, convulsions, menstrual cramps, infections, and a wide range of other ailments. Tinctures were manufactured by pharmaceutical companies like Bayer and Parke-Davis.[9] By the turn of the century, there were hundreds of cannabis preparations listed in the *United States Pharmacopeia*.

RACISM AND THE CANNABIS CRACKDOWN

In the 1920s and '30s, fascism was on the rise, and racial intolerance was a cornerstone of that philosophy. Additionally, especially in the United States, there was a shift away from being a nation of farmers to becoming an industrial powerhouse. With this massive change occurring, people became fearful, and governments, for various reasons, often channeled that fear into racial prejudice.

In the United States, an enterprising young bureaucrat named Harry Anslinger, head of the newly formed Bureau of Narcotics, was looking for a way to grow his fledgling agency and seized on fear and racial prejudice as his tools. He teamed up with elected officials in the South who saw the black population and Mexican immigrants as a threat. These populations used an odd herb they called marijuana. Some local municipalities had outlawed this substance and used the laws to arrest blacks and Mexican people. Anslinger took that approach nationally and began an epic crusade to eradicate marijuana across the land in order to "save" unsuspecting white adolescents from this scourge. Anslinger wrote the Marijuana Tax Act of 1937, which effectively stopped the use of cannabis as medicine and began America's long "war on drugs."

In the late 1960s, the Anslinger approach of drug policy based on skin color was ratcheted upward by the Nixon administration's official War on Drugs. Black people in particular were targeted for arrest, and the result has been massively lopsided incarceration figures when it comes to drug offenses. According to ACLU Policy Analyst Charlotte Resing, "People in the United States use and sell marijuana at roughly the same rate regardless of their race, yet a Black person is almost

TESTIMONIAL: IT WORKED FOR ME

My condition before CBD was intolerable. As a result of Poland syndrome (underdeveloped chest muscles), I had constant pain exacerbated by age and arthritis. I could not turn my head to the left. The pain led to insomnia and a high level of anxiety.

I had turned to prescription medication for pain relief and sleep, which quickly wreaked havoc on my digestive tract. A friend and my daughter encouraged me to try a CBD tincture and topical salve. The very first day I felt better. I had hope! Over the next few months I adjusted and readjusted dosage, timing, and ratio. I was able to stop the prescription medication completely.

It is a process that will never be completely stationary. I am not cured of my lifelong deformity, and there are occasional flare-ups of pain and inflammation. So, I adjust the CBD. But I am now in control, I am comfortable, I have more flexibility in my neck, and I am sleeping. I feel very grateful that CBD works for me.

Ginny C.

74 YEARS OLD, VENICE, FL

four times more likely than a white person to be arrested for marijuana possession nationwide."[10]

This use of racism as a drug policy tool seems, at last, to be coming to a close, in part because the public is now far more knowledgeable about cannabis and its components, like CBD.

How Does CBD Work?

How exactly the CBD molecule acts in the body is not entirely understood. However, the simplified version is this: When any drug enters the body, it stimulates receptors, ion channels, enzymes, and protein transporters. We know that the body has natural receptors for cannabis. Two such receptors have been identified thus far: CB1 and CB2. CBD can bind to either of these receptors. When CBD binds with those receptors, it is functioning as part of the endocannabinoid system (ECS).

If you would like a more detailed explanation, ProjectCBD.org has an excellent explanation of the complex process behind CBD's ability to assist with pain reduction and other aspects of treating disease.

THE ENDOCANNABINOID SYSTEM

The ECS was discovered in the early 1990s. Given how important it is to our well-being, it is amazing that it was not discovered earlier, but the federal prohibition of cannabis made research difficult. With this late discovery of the ECS, we can see a concrete example of how costly the prohibition has been in terms of our knowledge. As Project CBD states on its website, "The discovery of receptors in the brain that respond pharmacologically to cannabis—and the subsequent identification of endogenous cannabinoid compounds in our own bodies that bind to these receptors—has significantly advanced our understanding of human biology, health, and disease."[11]

Precisely how the endocannabinoid system works is very complex and not completely known. However, the purpose of the ECS can be simply stated: It aids the body in maintaining physiological balance.

The body's major organs have cannabis receptors, and these organs make up two of the key elements in physiological balance: the endocrine and the nervous systems.

It is important to remember that the body itself creates cannabinoid-like substances that work with the ECS. There are two identified internal cannabinoids: anandamide and 2-AG. When some part of the body is out of balance, the ECS will increase the number of internal cannabinoids and direct them to certain receptors to help return the body to a balanced state. But sometimes the body cannot create enough of these internal cannabinoids, and that is when cannabis can be helpful.

RESEARCH ON CBD'S EFFECTIVENESS

The discovery of the ECS was a major scientific breakthrough, and scientists were quick to understand the implications of this newly revealed physiological system. Research accelerated at an enormous

CHART 1: CBD Research 1991–2019

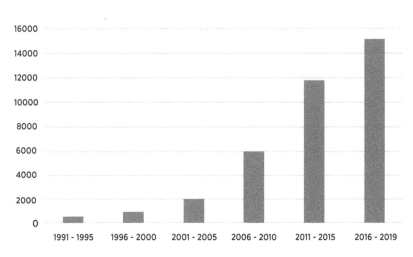

Number of scientific studies that mention CBD

rate. Research into CBD was particularly favored because of its multiple interactions with the human body and its minimal psychoactivity. In 1990, the year before announcement of the ECS discovery, there were just 94 articles that mentioned cannabidiol in the scientific literature. But as you can see in chart 1, scientific articles mentioning CBD have gone through the roof, with 15,200 articles between 2016 and 2019.[12]

This level of research is truly exciting for the patient contemplating or currently employing CBD. In 2019 alone there have been published studies on CBD and Parkinson's,[13] anxiety and sleep disorders,[14] chronic pain,[15] and more.

Side Effects of CBD

Clearly a drug that can treat so many diseases and illnesses must have profound effects on the human body. Thankfully most of those effects are targeted at the illness being treated, but if you are contemplating CBD use or are already using it, you need to be aware that CBD, as with any medication or pharmaceutical, can have some side effects, particularly at high doses. Cannabis clinicians always advise patients to "start low and go slow." Common side effects include drowsiness, lethargy, change in mood, dry mouth, diarrhea, appetite changes, and dizziness.

Some headlines recently warned of "liver toxicity" associated with CBD.[16] There are reasons to be concerned when taking large doses of CBD, such as those prescribed to patients taking the FDA-approved CBD medicine Epidiolex (normally 20 mg/kg, or almost 1,100 mg a day for a 120-pound adult). These doses are much higher than those normally needed, however, and there is no reason to believe that CBD warrants any more attention than other drugs when it comes to liver health.

Chronic Pain and Anxiety

Patients living with chronic pain may often experience anxiety as well. In a 2013 study that screened patients with chronic pain, it was found that 45 percent had one or more common anxiety disorders. These same patients reported significantly worse pain and health-related quality of life than patients without anxiety.[17] Another study points to as many as 80 percent of pain patients experiencing anxiety and depression.[18]

At one time it was thought that anxiety and depression in chronic pain patients were psychological rather than biological, but new research into how the brain works has discovered that pain "shares some biological mechanisms with anxiety and depression."[19] This overlap of pain and anxiety is particularly prevalent in fibromyalgia and irritable bowel syndrome as well as chronic low back pain, neuropathic pain, and headaches.

Treatment of pain-related anxiety can be complex. Powerful psychiatric medications are often prescribed, but increasingly doctors prefer to recommend nondrug therapies such as exercise and relaxation training.

CBD can be effective medication for pain-related anxiety, relieving both the pain and anxiety associated with it. CBD's well-known neuroprotectant properties may play an important role in this two-for-one therapeutic effect.[20] Patients who have successfully employed CBD to treat pain will often state they feel "less anxious" (see "Testimonial: It Worked for Me," page 21).

DRUG INTERACTIONS

If you are thinking about using CBD to treat one of the illnesses listed in this book (see chapter 3), then you are probably already using conventional prescribed medications. You are also probably aware that drugs can interact with one another to minimize or maximize a desired effect. It is important to be aware of possible drug interactions with CBD and your regular medications. The CBD Interaction with Commonly Prescribed Drugs chart (see page 116) provides helpful information about possible drug interactions between CBD and many prescribed medications.

CBD and the Law

CBD's popularity stems in large part from its nonintoxicating properties, but the other obvious reason is the drug's availability. Unlike its notorious molecular cousin THC, which remains illegal on the federal level, CBD derived from hemp is legal in nearly all the United States and can even be purchased online. CBD derived from cannabis plants (as opposed to hemp plants) is still classified by the federal government in Schedule I.

IS CBD LEGAL?

The short answer is yes, but in the complex world of cannabis it is important to know that "yes" comes with some caveats.

Medical cannabis is complicated and confusing. More than 30 state laws legalize access to medical cannabis, and another 11 have legalized adult recreational access to cannabis, but federal law says that any access to cannabis is illegal. So, which is true, and what is legal?

Recall that CBD can be obtained from the cannabis plant and from hemp plants, and therein lies the trick. Hemp is legal in the United States. For many years there were just a few states where hemp was legal. The 2014 Farm Bill changed things by allowing institutions of higher learning and state agricultural departments to grow hemp if state law permitted. The 2014 Farm Bill also standardized the THC content of industrial hemp at 0.3 percent. This had several beneficial consequences for CBD, especially for research. Several state institutions of higher learning embraced hemp as a way to accelerate cannabis research (remember, hemp is still part of the cannabis family).

In 2018 the US Congress expanded the Farm Bill significantly by removing hemp from the list of controlled substances and including hemp as a commodity that could be covered by crop insurance. Some states rejected the 2018 Farm Bill and outlawed hemp; however, the majority of states moved forward with including hemp in agricultural programs. Many new hemp farmers began cultivating the plant to extract CBD, and thus the number of CBD products began to grow.

CBD AND DRUG TESTING

Many people work at jobs where they are subject to random or routine drug testing. This is true even in states with full medical cannabis access. If you have a job that requires drug tests, you may want to think twice about using CBD, including CBD extracted from hemp. Even though hemp has just 0.3 percent THC, and your CBD claims to have no THC at all, there could be trace amounts of THC that, over time, could build up in your system and trigger a positive urine test. Worse yet, not all CBD manufacturers have exacting standards when it comes to their products. A 2017 study found that some CBD had enough THC to cause users to easily fail drug tests.[21]

At least one study claims topical application of THC will not trigger a drug test,[22] so topical application of CBD may be safe. This does not apply to transdermal patches; even CBD-only patches may have enough THC to build up over time. Therefore, if you are subject to random drug tests, you should probably avoid CBD.

CBD Myths

We have covered a lot of ground in this chapter, but before we leave behind the basics of CBD, we should address some of the myths associated with this substance.

CBD is not psychoactive. You will hear that a lot, and it is simply a sloppy use of words. A better way to phrase it would be "CBD will not get you intoxicated." Like every medicine, CBD has some psychoactivity. For that matter, so does caffeine. Psychoactive means "affecting the mind," and any drug that enters the body has this potential. But do not think CBD will get you stoned. That will not happen.

CBD is a sedative. For some people at some doses, CBD can be sedating, but many others say that CBD helps them be more alert. Cannabis compounds are biphasic, which means that low and high doses can create opposite effects. This is why it is very important to start low and go slow. Take the time to learn how your body responds to CBD.

CBD is legal everywhere. This is one of the most confusing aspects of CBD. Federal law, which still claims cannabis has no accepted medical value, really muddies the water here. The DEA will tell you that CBD is illegal, but many state laws have a different opinion. The 2018 Farm Bill legalized hemp and removed it from the controlled substances list. CBD, as we know, can be extracted from hemp. Whether to use CBD is a very personal decision for you to make. Some people, no matter what, will never break any law. For others, there comes a point at which they believe federal law has not kept pace with science. Several major corporations, including CVS and Walgreens, have made the decision that hemp-based CBD is legal, and you can now find products on their shelves.

TESTIMONIAL: IT WORKED FOR ME

I am an oncology nurse turned patient. Four years ago, I suddenly found myself in a wheelchair with 90 percent of my small nerve fibers destroyed. I had severe head-to-toe neuropathy, painful allodynia, and constant neuropathic itch. My left brain was being attacked by an unidentified autoimmune component. I lived at a pain level from eight to ten and could no longer work. Whatever was attacking my brain also caused severe visual problems, and driving became a terrifying and dangerous experience.

But from the very first drops of a full-spectrum CBD tincture, that changed. I am now able to enjoy life with a pain level average of two, and I only occasionally have neuropathic itch or allodynia.

I use a CBD and THC tincture (roughly 5.5 mg of each) for my daily medicine, as I find I need both to address all of my medical issues and to maintain a low pain level. If I were forced to choose just one, I believe I would choose the CBD, provided it was a full-spectrum, clean variety. THC did not help with my visual problems. I find CBD gives me great relief in terms of any pain caused by inflammation. It also gives me a nice sense of calm that I was not expecting.

Elizabeth H.

55 YEARS OLD, MIAMI, FL

HOW TO USE THIS BOOK

This book is designed to be a helpful guide on the use of CBD—whether for yourself, a loved one, or even a pet. Our focus is pain relief, and for that reason we have chosen to highlight only those ailments that have pain associated with them (see chapter 3). CBD is remarkably versatile, and there are other ailments that respond well to it. There are also numerous reference sources on CBD that cover these other illnesses. We encourage you to learn as much as you can about this remarkable compound as well as other parts of the cannabis plant. At the back of the book, you will find a Resources list to help you learn more.

Now that you have read about the basics, it is time to move on to specifics. You can approach this in any way with which you are most comfortable. You may want to skip to chapter 3 and learn how CBD can help the specific ailment that afflicts you or a loved one. Or you may want to continue to chapter 2 and learn about the various CBD products that are out there and how to find the correct product just for you. CBD has taken the country by storm, and there are some unscrupulous manufacturers wanting to make a buck. Be aware of that, but do not worry. We will help guide you to CBD products that are safe and effective.

CHAPTER TWO

YOUR CBD PRODUCT PRIMER

Now that we have covered some of the basics of CBD, it is time to look at the CBD marketplace, which may very well prove to be the most confusing aspect of your CBD experience. This chapter describes CBD products that are available, the pros and cons of each type, and information to help you choose a quality medication. It will walk you through where to buy CBD and help you sort through the myriad of products and information.

A Note of Caution

You have made the decision to try CBD. Or perhaps you are already using CBD but need some guidance in finding the right product. That is the purpose of this chapter. We want to help you find a product that is safe, high quality, and easy to acquire on a continuing basis.

But we especially want you to be safe. It is likely that you or someone you love is in pain and suffering from one of the 21 ailments we cover in this book (see chapter 3). These are complex ailments and require the attention of a doctor, nurse, or other healthcare professional. We encourage you to discuss CBD with the members of your healthcare team because many of these illnesses have a wide variety and large number of prescribed medications, and you want to be certain there are no harmful interactions. Chapter 3 provides information on drug interactions, but no book can take the place of a clinician's opinion.

It can be hard to discuss CBD with your doctor because of the stigma attached to anything having to do with cannabis or even natural remedies. Fortunately, the attitudes of physicians are changing as they, too, become educated about the endogenous cannabinoid system.

Where to Shop

Perhaps the most amazing thing about shopping for CBD is that you can do so from the comfort of your home. Most CBD product manufacturers provide online shopping at their websites. At the back of this book you will find a section called Recommended CBD Brands that can lead you to many of these reputable companies.

What about Amazon? Well, search for "CBD oil" at Amazon and you might be overwhelmed by the choices. However, these products are actually hemp oil, not CBD extract. In fact, Amazon prohibits sale of any products with cannabidiol (CBD)[23] but does not prohibit searches using the term "CBD." This should give you a good idea of how the market has blurred the lines between hemp oil and CBD.

Finally, if you live in a state with a medical cannabis law (or full legalization), you can visit a dispensary to look for and acquire products, although depending upon the state, you may need a doctor's recommendation to enter the dispensary.

HEMP-DERIVED CBD VS. HEMP OIL

Amazon's array of CBD products brings us to a very important discussion: the differences between hemp-derived CBD and hemp oil.

The 2018 Farm Bill, discussed in chapter 1, created a huge "green rush" that is continuing to develop and expand. Hemp is now legal to grow in any state, and products manufactured from hemp can be sold throughout the United States.

Hemp oil, as opposed to CBD oil, is derived from the stalks and seeds of the hemp plant. It has been available for years in health food stores, where people would purchase it as a food supplement. It is very high in antioxidants, omega-3, and omega-6 but contains a miniscule amount of CBD. Hemp oil is made by pressing the hemp seeds and stalks to obtain the oil.

To achieve any therapeutic benefit, you must obtain CBD that is extracted from the leaves of the hemp plant using a solvent and distillation process. There are several processes for CBD extraction, and those who are interested can find plenty of websites that explain the various options for extracting CBD.

In years past it would require an enormous amount of hemp leaves to extract CBD, and it was not a particularly efficient or economical process. With the recent CBD "green rush," efforts have been underway to get more bang for the buck. This has entailed modifying the hemp plant to manufacture more CBD while still retaining the THC at less than 0.3 percent. These efforts will continue as long as cannabis remains illegal under federal law.

TESTIMONIAL: IT WORKED FOR ME

I have always had trouble with sleep and anxiety issues. About two years ago, my neurologist recommended a tincture with CBD and THC. I live in Florida, which has a medical cannabis law, but acquiring a medical card was very expensive, and I thought I would try CBD first to see if it worked. I watched a lot of YouTube videos about CBD, and eventually I ordered CBD online, and it has helped with pain and anxiety. Then a friend told me about SRQ Botanicals, a local shop that sells only CBD products. I liked having a store to go to and people to speak with about the use of CBD. Everyone who works there seems very knowledgeable. I was able to buy CBD with a higher concentration than what I was getting online, and that has been helpful and is more economical.

Rosan Y.

72 YEARS OLD, SARASOTA, FL

CANNABIS-DERIVED CBD

For those who live in a medical cannabis or fully legalized state, there is another option for CBD products: cannabis-derived CBD. This means that the CBD is extracted from a cannabis plant rather than hemp. It also means the CBD oil will have THC, although the THC may be at very minimal levels. These CBD oils are normally provided as tinctures with ratios of both compounds. So, for example, you might be able to obtain a 3:1 tincture, which means there are three parts of CBD to one part of THC. There are many different ratios available, some as high as 18:1. In oils with this high level of CBD, the intoxicating effects of THC will be neutralized by the CBD, but THC will still contribute to the overall therapeutic effect. As you will learn in chapter 3, there are some diseases that benefit from the addition of a small amount of THC.

Cannabis-derived CBD is far more efficient and economical. Without the restraint of keeping THC at less than 0.3 percent, which hobbles the hemp farmer, a cannabis farmer can manipulate his or her plants to produce higher amounts of CBD than would normally be produced.

The Right Product for You

As you begin your search for the right CBD product, there are several considerations that will affect your decision. You will discover there are numerous delivery methods, including tinctures, topical preparations, vape pens, transdermal patches, capsules, and edibles. Regardless of delivery method, however, there are considerations that factor into every decision. Some of these factors are simple and straightforward, such as cost. Others will call on you to make a personal decision, and it may take a couple of different tries before finding the CBD therapy that is right for you. Factors for consideration include:

Full-Spectrum or Isolate: As you read the labels or packaging information for the CBD products, these terms will likely appear. Basically, they refer to the final product of the extraction process. An isolate CBD product undergoes a process that extracts just the CBD molecules in isolation and then puts those molecules of CBD into a carrier medium of some sort: oil, salve, etc. In full-spectrum CBD, the extraction process captures the CBD as well as other cannabinoids, terpenes, and compounds. These additional compounds contribute to the entourage effect, which is a theory that cannabinoid compounds work more effectively together rather than in isolation. There is no universally right or wrong choice, and patients will need to experiment to determine which product works best for them.

Concentration: CBD can come in many forms. A concentrate is a high-potency CBD oil. Concentrates may be referred to as wax, shatter, rosin, and FECO (full extract cannabis oil). These products allow patients to consume large dosages of CBD. The potency of a concentrate ranges from 20 percent to over 70 percent. The potency of the concentration varies depending on what part of the plant was used to process the oil. Stalks and stems will produce only small amounts of CBD, leaves have more, and the flowers, or cola, will contain the most CBD. Unfortunately, concentrates are difficult to measure. Since most people tend to eyeball the amount they are consuming, accuracy of the dose is nearly impossible.

Speed and Duration: The manner in which the CBD product is used will determine the speed and duration of the effect. Inhalation remains the most rapid way to introduce cannabinoids into the human body. CBD vape pens can provide rapid onset of relief, but that relief may be short-lived compared to CBD capsules, which take time to digest and enter the system but have a longer period of effect. For those who may be concerned about the effects of CBD, transdermal patches offer an interesting benefit because they can be removed, and the drug effects will dissipate in about 20 minutes. When treating pain, you may discover that a combination of delivery methods is preferable—for example, capsules for systemic relief, with a vape pen used to treat breakthrough pain.

Ease and Familiarity: If you are new to CBD, you may have initial feelings of anxiety as you navigate your way through this unfamiliar territory. This is natural. It is important to remember that CBD is safe and nonintoxicating. Delivery methods have vastly improved, and you no longer must smoke CBD in order to obtain relief. If you prefer taking pills, you will find CBD capsules available in varying doses. Tinctures are another option. As you learn more about CBD, this will all become easier.

Flavor: This is an area that few people initially think of, but it can have a huge impact on how you feel about a product. Not too long ago, before the CBD boom gathered steam, CBD oil was a bit like classic ice cream, with one flavor: vanilla. CBD oil tasted a lot like hemp, which is to say it tasted like mown grass. Some people did not mind, but others were repulsed. As the market began to grow, entrepreneurs realized that flavor was an issue and became more inventive. Currently, many CBD products have flavors such as mint, citrus, and berry. It is important to recognize that most flavored CBD tinctures are made with CBD isolate, not full-spectrum CBD. Manufacturers of full-spectrum CBD have modified their formularies in recent years, and high-quality CBD tinctures now have a more neutral flavor.

Cost: For most of us, cost is a consideration. Insurance will not cover the costs of CBD medication, so if you decide on CBD therapy, the costs will be out-of-pocket. This is where understanding the difference between hemp oil and hemp-derived CBD oil is of vital importance. Hemp oil will be significantly cheaper but has no therapeutic benefit because it has no CBD. Exploring your options is important, but do not get fooled into buying hemp oil disguised as CBD oil.

Delivery Methods for CBD

There are essentially four ways to use CBD for medical purposes: oral, inhalation, topical/transdermal, and suppository. Each has its advantages. See the chart CBD Product Considerations at a Glance on page 36 for a summary of product availability.

ORAL INGESTION

CBD can be orally ingested via four methods: capsules, tinctures, edibles, or pastes and concentrates.

CBD Drinks

CBD is literally everywhere! There are dozens of brands of CBD water, infused sodas, teas (kombucha is a big hit in this category), and beer. Until a few years ago, such concoctions would have been unthinkable because the theory was that cannabinoids could be dissolved only in oil. But new extraction methods have allowed manufacturers to dissolve CBD in water, which has led to these new delivery forms. From a therapeutic delivery perspective, these drinks really are not an option. There are stability issues, and the CBD can leave the liquid and cling to the container's interior. While this is not the best scenario for someone seeking pain relief, CBD drinks can be a refreshing source of hydration and provide another way to feed your ECS system and contribute to an overall sense of well-being.

Capsules: Capsules are familiar, and many people choose capsule form for their CBD. The advantage of capsules is the familiarity of the method and the fact that they will act systemically, delivering a measured dose of CBD to the entire body. Capsules come in many different strengths, and new users should find the lowest strength available. Costs are equally broad, ranging from $25 for 60 5-mg capsules from bluebirdbotanicals.com to $120 for 60 18-mg capsules at Charlottesweb.com. See Recommended CBD Brands at the back of this book for other manufacturers.

Tinctures: The ongoing renaissance of cannabis as medicine has reignited interest in tinctures, which were once a staple for physicians even as late as the mid-20th century. Today's entrepreneurs researched original preparations of cannabis in old pharmacopeias and developed modern CBD tinctures based on those preparations. Tinctures can be alcohol or oil based, with oil-based tinctures taking longer for onset (see chart 2, page 36). Tinctures have many advantages. Taken properly (hold the drops under the tongue and let them absorb), they can be very fast acting. They are discreet and easy to transport. They can be very effective for breakthrough pain. Use caution, and be sure you are getting hemp-derived CBD, not hemp oil. CBD tinctures run a broad gamut in price. You might need your math cap to determine which are the best buys because each website seems to provide different measurements, from ounces to grams, and at different prices. Costs can range from $60 for a half ounce at one website to $139 for 30 ml at another. However, when converting the measurements, these are approximately the same price. Suggestion: Siri or Alexa can be a big help in converting ounces to milliliters or milligrams to grams.

Edibles: People are intrigued with cannabinoid edibles, and there are, of course, CBD edibles. For those who hate to take pills or tinctures, edibles may be a fun way to take medicine. After all, there are adult gummy daily vitamins and supplements. So, if you are taking CBD strictly as a supplement, the edible format may not be bad. In fact, it may ensure that you take the CBD every day. The problem with edibles as a medicinal delivery form is the production, which may not be up to the same standards as those employed by tincture and capsule manufacturers. And gummies are likely to have sugar, which may be a serious problem for some. Additionally, anything you ingest takes longer to reach your bloodstream, and the times can be erratic depending on what else you may have ingested.

Pastes and Concentrates: Depending on how much CBD you require on an ongoing basis, concentrates or pastes may be an appropriate option for you. These delivery forms can be obtained with CBD content varying from 45 percent to almost 90 percent. This allows for a more economical administration of CBD but requires more active involvement of the patient in terms of preparation and administration.

INHALATION

The iconic image of someone smoking a joint to get medical relief from cannabis is still prevalent, but like just about everything else, modern technology has provided new answers to old methods.

Vaporizer Pen or E-Cigarette

The term vaporizer pen (more commonly referred to as a "vape pen") and e-cigarette are often used interchangeably, but e-cigs are more associated with tobacco smokers. Vape pens allow the user to purchase "pods" that fit on the rechargeable pen. Vaping is much easier on the throat and lungs than smoking a joint. With vaping there is minimal smoke, and it is cooler in temperature and has little to no odor. Many CBD manufacturers will arrange partnerships with vape pen manufacturers so as to simplify pod production. Only buy vape products from reputable manufacturers (see How to Use a Vape Pen, page 35).

How to Use a Vape Pen

If you have never used a vape pen, you need not worry. Manufacturers have ensured that they are easy to use, and of course there are numerous websites and YouTube videos that may be of assistance.

Disposable vape pens are available at various CBD product sites and might be a good way to start. They cost around $20.

Nearly all vape pens, even some disposable ones, are rechargeable. Disposable models will have just one pod, but other vape pens have interchangeable pods. Most vape pens have an activation button that you press to heat the oil in the pod, while some require that you initiate the inhalation process. In either case, the heating element works very fast, delivering a stream of vapor that delivers CBD to your lungs, where it is absorbed very quickly into your bloodstream.

Caution: Be certain that you purchase your CBD vape product from a reputable manufacturer. Avoid products that are combined with vitamin E, propylene glycol (PEG or PG), or flavoring additives. These can increase the chance of contamination.

CHART 2: CBD Product Considerations at a Glance

	CONCENTRATION	SPEED	DURATION
TINCTURE	2.5 to 5 mg	15 minutes to an hour. Oil-based tinctures may take 1 to 2 hours.	6 to 8 hours
CAPSULES	5 mg and up	1 to 2 hours	6 hours
EDIBLES/DRINKS	Normally around 10 mg per edible	1 to 2 hours	6 to 8 hours
VAPE PEN	Variable—2 mg and up	Very rapid onset—a few minutes	2 to 3 hours
TOPICAL	Large variety of concentrations ranging from 100 mg to 500 mg of CBD per container	10 to 20 minutes	Several hours—very depen-dent on site and patient's overall physical condition
TRANSDERMAL	10 mg per patch	20 minutes	8 to 12 hours
SUPPOSITORY	25 to 50 mg per unit	15 to 30 minutes	1 to 3 hours

EASE OF USE	FLAVOR	COST
Moderate	Affected by the oil in which the CBD is suspended	$25 and ↑ depending on size of bottle and manufacturing
Good	N/A	$30 and ↑ depending on quantity and dose
Good	A vast variety	$10 and ↑
Moderate	N/A	$20 and ↑ Disposables are an inexpensive way to become acquainted.
Good	N/A	$16 and ↑
Good	N/A	$12 to $20 depending on potency
Moderate to difficult	N/A	Availability is sketchy and price variable—$50 for 10 on one site

TOPICAL/TRANSDERMAL

CBD salves are a wonderful delivery method for localized pain such as arthritis or neuropathic pain. There are creams that have a smooth texture and salves that are more formidable. Deciding which to use is a personal choice. Some have menthol added, making them similar to Bengay. Simply apply the salve to your aching muscles or joints. Transdermal patches are applied to the skin, and the CBD is absorbed into your body. The effects can last for 8 to 12 hours.

SUPPOSITORIES

A fairly new entry on the CBD market is the CBD suppository. There is very little clinical research about this delivery form, and rectal bioavailability has its skeptics. Nevertheless, this option is available and could be useful in some situations, such as end-of-life care or when certain diseases such as ALS, MS, and cancer become advanced to the point of rendering a patient incapable of ingesting or inhaling CBD.

How to Identify High-Quality CBD

It cannot be said often enough: All CBD is not alike. The market is unregulated, so it is advised to proceed with caution. Know your product!

INGREDIENTS

The first thing to look for is a listing of ingredients on the label. If there is no list of ingredients, then it would be best to avoid purchasing that or any product from the labeled company. The number one thing to look for on the label is the phrase "hemp-derived CBD." Hemp oil is not the same as CBD oil. The label should specify "hemp-derived CBD," or it may even say "cannabis sativa (<0.3%)." Beware of any product label that makes a specific claim of being able to "cure" or "heal."

BRAND TRANSPARENCY

Whether you buy online or in one of the many CBD shops that have been popping up, you want to look for brand transparency. A transparent CBD company will not hesitate to share information about the product, and that information should be immediately available. Do not trust a salesperson's response of "Oh, I can get that for you. What's your email?" Because the CBD market is largely unregulated, there are no nationwide rules for what should be on a product label, but here are a few things to look for:

Amount of CBD in the Item and Serving Size

Normally this will be found in an obvious position on the label. It will typically read something like "600 mg," which indicates the total concentration of CBD in the container. If you are buying tincture, capsules, suppositories, or patches, there should be information on the dose per unit. It will say something like "60 capsules with 10 mg CBD each."

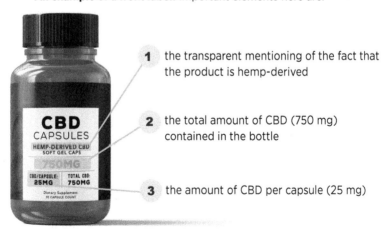

An example of a front label. Important elements here are:

1 the transparent mentioning of the fact that the product is hemp-derived

2 the total amount of CBD (750 mg) contained in the bottle

3 the amount of CBD per capsule (25 mg)

An example of a back label. Important elements here are:

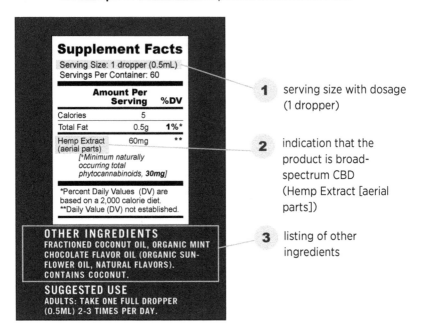

Supplement Facts

Serving Size: 1 dropper (0.5mL)
Servings Per Container: 60

	Amount Per Serving	%DV
Calories	5	
Total Fat	0.5g	**1%***
Hemp Extract (aerial parts)	60mg	**
[*Minimum naturally occurring total phytocannabinoids, **30mg**]		

*Percent Daily Values (DV) are based on a 2,000 calorie diet.
**Daily Value (DV) not established.

OTHER INGREDIENTS
FRACTIONED COCONUT OIL, ORGANIC MINT CHOCOLATE FLAVOR OIL (ORGANIC SUNFLOWER OIL, NATURAL FLAVORS). CONTAINS COCONUT.

SUGGESTED USE
ADULTS: TAKE ONE FULL DROPPER (0.5ML) 2-3 TIMES PER DAY.

1 serving size with dosage (1 dropper)

2 indication that the product is broad-spectrum CBD (Hemp Extract [aerial parts])

3 listing of other ingredients

Batch Number

Batch or lot number provides the means to access the lab test, and, ideally, one can go to the product website and download the lab test. This is something you are more likely to find in states with medical cannabis laws or on products that come from states with medical cannabis laws. Sometimes it will be found stamped on the bottom of the container.

Product Testing

The batch or lot number will lead you to the lab report (or COA—certificate of analysis), which has an enormous amount of data. The information listed will typically include percentage of CBD and other cannabinoids, terpenes (compounds that contribute to the aroma of cannabis), heavy metal screening, pesticide screening, and solvent screening. It is not necessary for you to understand all of these, but it is important that a company provide the analysis.

COST

The cost of the product does not indicate the quality. Indeed, it is quite the opposite in some cases. Keep in mind that the market is unregulated, and there are charlatans who will gladly charge you 10 times what a product is worth.

Using CBD for the First Time

You have made a product selection and are now ready to use CBD for the first time. If you have used cannabis in the past, you are probably comfortable with using CBD without any reservations. But if you have never used cannabis, aka marijuana, then you may be a bit nervous. This is understandable because of the previously discussed stigma and misinformation. However, you need not be nervous. CBD will not intoxicate you, and there is no high. Just remember, start low and go slow. In other words, start with a low dose and increase slowly.

DECIDING ON A DOSE

Most CBD products such as tinctures and capsules will have recommended doses on the label or packaging. If you have never taken cannabinoids before, you may want to start with half the recommended dose. When taking capsules, always start with one a day for three to five days just to see what effect they may have. Sometimes the other ingredients in capsules can cause complications such as diarrhea.

WHAT TO EXPECT

Every one of us has a different biological makeup, varying levels of enzymes, hormones, chemicals, and even natural cannabinoids known as anandamide and 2-AG. Because CBD will directly interact with your endocannabinoid system (ECS), which, in turn, will affect

A Budget Saver's Buying Guide

As you have learned, buying CBD can be daunting. Move slowly and deliberately to find the product that is best for you. Here are some tips to do so:

1. Determine which form of CBD is best for you—oral, inhaled, or topical—and focus on that method. Do not let yourself be distracted by online ads or "helpful" CBD store merchants who try to steer you toward another method of administration.

2. Use the Internet to comparison shop. Even if you plan to buy your CBD locally, it does not hurt to shop around, and the Internet is an easy way to do so.

3. If it seems too good to be true, it probably is. This is an old maxim but a very helpful one when shopping for CBD. Beware of products or websites that use the words cure and heal.

4. Look for companies that offer sample-size product so you can try a product before investing a significant amount of money.

5. Compare apples to apples. In other words, try to standard-ize the offerings. One company may list 30 ml of tincture. Another may say 1 ounce. They are the same thing. Alexa or Siri can be a big help with conversion math, or you can make use of www.asknumbers.com.

6. If you are buying online, identify a product and company you like and then research the company. Spend some time doing different searches about the XYZ CBD Co., and see what is being said about it on the Web.

7. It is okay to say, "No thanks." If you are undecided or uncom-fortable, just say no. There are numerous franchise CBD stores that often offer just one product line of CBD. Do not purchase simply because you are there and the clerk seems nice. Do your homework!

TESTIMONIAL: IT WORKED FOR ME

I am a two-time breast cancer survivor first diagnosed at age 43 and then again at 45. I was introduced to cannabis during my second cancer battle in 2013. Prior to that I had no knowledge of cannabis in any form. I was allergic to all the antiemetics, and I was emaciated, nauseous, severely constipated, and fatigued. Cannabis changed all that.

I have used cannabis in many different ways: edibles, vaping, smoking, topicals, tinctures, and oils. My preferred method is a transdermal patch that has a 1:1 combination of CBD:THC. I am very sensitive to THC, and it makes me paranoid. But in my experience, if I keep the ratio of THC to CBD equal or the CBD greater (for example, 2:12 THC:CBD), then I do not experience the negative side effects of paranoia and crippling anxiety. I do not use pharmaceuticals anymore except for my inhalers for my asthma.

Nique

51 YEARS OLD, FALL RIVER, MA

those enzymes, hormones, and chemicals, it is almost impossible to say how you will be affected by CBD. Some report an almost immediate sense of well-being. For others it can be a more measured response. Some patients have reported that they suddenly realize they feel better. CBD will not interfere with your activities of daily life, so do the things you would normally do and let the CBD do its job.

MAKE DOSAGE ADJUSTMENTS

As time moves on and you continue your CBD use, it may become necessary to make dosage adjustments. How will you know? By listening to your body. If there is one dramatic difference between cannabinoid therapy and conventional medicine, it is the active participation of the patient. This is one reason that keeping notes is particularly helpful. Dosage adjustments are normal at the start of CBD therapy, and once you reach a good level, things may be fine for weeks or months, but with time you may notice the CBD is not quite as effective as it once was. At that point you may want to increase your dose. Once again, go slow. Some people have also found that discontinuing CBD for one or two days and then restarting helps reset the ECS.

CBD for Pets

It turns out that all mammals have an ECS, including your pets. So, it is only natural to wonder if CBD could help your dog or cat. The answer is yes.

Fundamentally, humans, canines, and felines are extremely similar. We have similar internal organs, and thus our pets can contract painful illnesses, too. As a result, people have had great success with using CBD and other cannabis products on their pets.

EFFECTIVENESS IN PETS

Just as it is with humans, CBD's effectiveness in treating pets varies. To date, there is very little specific research that has been conducted on the effectiveness of CBD in treating dog and cat illnesses. Another complication is communication—our pets cannot accurately tell us how they are feeling and whether CBD is helping them feel better. So, it becomes extra important to monitor pets carefully after starting CBD therapy. Just as we start low and go slow in humans, we should do the same with pets.

Some applications of CBD in pets will be easy to observe. Many people use CBD to treat a pet's anxiety, especially with respect to thunderstorms or fireworks. Effectiveness in these situations is easy to assess. Similarly, if your pet has arthritis and you treat it with CBD, you may notice an improvement in how they are able to move their sore joints. For more serious ailments such as epilepsy, stroke, or even cancer, it can be hard to measure reactions. Once again, a notebook is recommended to record doses and reactions.

DELIVERY METHODS FOR PETS

CBD delivery methods are similar in pets with the exception of vape pens. Some might be inclined to use a vape pen and then administer the CBD by blowing in the pet's face. The reaction will almost certainly be for the pet to withdraw. Pets have highly sensitive olfactory senses, and it is easy to overload them. Please refrain from using this delivery method with your pet.

Tinctures are easy to administer. Just add the tincture to your pet's food or squirt it directly into your pet's mouth. Either method will result in the loss of some CBD. There are also CBD treats for pets that are safe and easy to administer.

Topical use is effective, but only if applied directly to the skin. For daily dosing, use the inside of the ear, where skin is easily accessible and where it is hard for the animal to lick the oil or salve off. CBD may be effective for skin rashes, but you will need to keep the animal from licking the area.

DOSAGE FOR PETS

If you purchase pet-specific CBD, the packaging will likely have recommendations with regard to dosing. Once again, start low and go slow. You may want to cut in half the recommended dose and build up to it over a week's time. In this way you will be able to judge if the CBD is having any negative effects on the animal. While there is some controversy about proper dosage, on average, most pet products recommend 1 to 5 mg per pound a day. In chapter 4 you will find a helpful chart that provides dosing per size of your pet. Once you determine

Hemp-Derived CBD Oil and Essential Oils

As you shop for CBD oil, whether for yourself or your pet, you may come across the term essential oils. Many CBD topicals and specifically prepared oils have essential oils listed on the ingredients label. What does that mean?

Well, it is a little muddied. Essential oils are compounds extracted from plants that provide aromatherapy for the user. Think of lavender, pine oil, citrus smells—all of these and many more are part of the essential oils. Normally, essential oils are not intended for oral consumption, so you will see them in CBD topical preparations or CBD aromatherapy diffusing preparations, which are promoted to help with energy, meditation, or sleep and require a diffusing machine.

There are products online that state they have CBD oil and essential oils mixed into a tincture for oral consumption. These essential oils are normally lemon, peppermint, or citrus and are added to improve taste. These are generally safe, but the use of the term essential oil does muddy the water a bit. If you decide to travel down the road of CBD with essential oils, be certain of the manufacturer's recommended methods of use and recognize that this particular form of CBD is designed more as a lifestyle supplement than as a therapeutic medication. There are a growing number of scientists and healthcare practitioners who advocate that we take better care of our ECS by employing these various methods. Just recognize that it may not provide the therapeutic relief you are seeking.

the dose, you will need to decide whether to divide the total dose into two servings or give the full dose once a day.

If you are using CBD to treat a pet's seizures, you will likely need much more than the recommended dose. Proceed slowly when treating such a serious ailment, and research online, preferably with comparisons by breed. With no clinical research to guide us, it is possible that high doses may be detrimental.

Keep It Simple

We are about to leave behind the basics of CBD and move on to applying CBD to specific ailments. We have covered a lot of ground, and you might be thinking, Good grief, this is too complex. But all beginnings are hard, and you are at the beginning of a new stage in treating your ailment. If you have one of the illnesses covered in the next chapter, then you are already very familiar with complex things. Somehow you have managed with all of that and still found your way to this point of considering a new medication. Well done!

The more you learn about CBD, the easier it will become. Just keep in mind why you are here and what you hope to gain from using CBD. You need to become an active participant in using this medicine, and that may be a new role for you, but it is a role that has the potential for huge dividends. If using CBD can help relieve your pain, isn't that worth doing a little extra homework?

PART II

CBD
RECOMMENDATIONS

CHAPTER THREE

CBD FOR PAINFUL CONDITIONS

In this chapter, you will learn about painful conditions that respond to CBD, some recommended dosing patterns, and possible drug interactions between CBD and conventional medications. Unlike some medications, CBD is not "one size fits all" when it comes to proper dosing. As we discussed in chapter 2, there are different forms of CBD (isolate and full-spectrum) and different delivery methods (oral, inhaled, topical) that can have a significant bearing on how to determine proper dosing.

Dosage Guidelines

There are many things to take into consideration when determining the proper dosing of CBD. Perhaps the most important aspect is flexibility. Your ECS is constantly in a state of flux and this has a bearing on proper dosing. Keep this in mind as you read the following sections on factors that influence dosing, and the important concept of starting low and going slow.

FACTORS THAT INFLUENCE DOSAGE

Regardless of which drugs you may use to treat your condition—CBD or others—there are numerous factors that influence proper dosing, including age, weight, sex, medication history, route of administration, and genetics. Your doctor takes these factors into consideration when writing your prescriptions, but now that you have decided to use CBD, you need to be aware of these factors as well.

Age: A critical factor in dosing is age. All drugs are metabolized, and our metabolism changes as we age. So, a 70-year-old may react differently to a medication than a 40-year-old. Children will obviously use lower doses because of their size and age, but elderly patients may also be candidates for lower dosing because they metabolize more slowly than an average adult.

Weight: It may seem obvious that an extremely thin person will require less of a drug than someone who is obese, but you may never have thought about this in relation to your own drug use. Normally your doctor and/or pharmacist factors in the body weight of a patient when preparing prescriptions. Often you will see this expressed as "milligram per kilogram," so the prescription may read something like "5 mg/kg." To figure a dose in this way, you need the patient's weight in kilograms (see chart 3 on page 58). Once you have ascertained the patient's kilogram weight, multiply the prescribed dose (in our example, 5 mg) by the kilogram weight. Dosing in this way can be extremely effective and is particularly useful when dosing cannabinoids.

Sex: Most drugs have the same effect on an individual regardless of their gender, but sex hormones can interfere with drug metabolism. Scientists are only just starting to understand this phenomenon. One important thing to remember is that most human research is conducted on healthy young males. An elderly female, for example, may react entirely differently.

Medication history: What other drugs are you taking? This is critical information that can have a very big impact on the effect of CBD. Some people turn to CBD in hopes of eliminating conventional medications, but you need to learn about those medications before eliminating them. Before you start CBD therapy, prepare a list of your current medications and a list of meds that you may have taken in the past. Perhaps start a small CBD notebook where you can list your current medications and keep track of your CBD dosing.

Route of administration: There are several routes of administration with any drug. With CBD the following routes are available: oral, sublingual (under the tongue), topical (administering directly to the skin), inhalation (vape pens), transdermal (patches that give a measured dose for a certain period of time), and suppositories (rectal or vaginal). The route you choose will depend on the disease or ailment you are treating. For example, a topical preparation may be more effective for an arthritis patient than taking a capsule.

Genetics: Increasingly, healthcare professionals are taking a patient's genetic makeup into account when prescribing medications or procedures. There is a field of research called pharmacogenomics (sometimes called pharmacogenetics) that studies how a person's genes affect how the person responds to medications. The Food and Drug Administration, which monitors drug safety in the United States, now includes pharmacogenomic information on the labels of almost

200 prescribed medications. As this field progresses, medicines will become more tailored to the patients and more effective.[24]

STARTING LOW

Start low and go slow. This is a phrase you will hear over and over when it comes to the medical use of cannabinoids, whether CBD or THC. Many people still have the mistaken impression that to use medical cannabis you must get high. Nothing could be further from the truth. There are some situations that require high dosing with THC and/or CBD. This is especially true when treating cancers. But this book is addressing the use of CBD, and you will see that low dosing, sometimes called *the Less Method,* is often effective. The Less Method chart on page 58 will give you an excellent starting point in using CBD.

WHEN TO START WITH A HIGH DOSE

Is there ever a time you should start with high doses of CBD? Most experts in the field would say no. But these same people will tell you there are times when you need to titrate the dose upward at a faster rate. Titrate refers to administering a drug in ever-increasing doses until the desired effect is obtained. Titration can refer to increasing the dose, the frequency of administration, or both.

Perhaps the best example of the need for higher doses of CBD with rapid titration can be found with pediatric epilepsy patients. Indeed, it was the case of young Charlotte Figi that first brought CBD to the nation's attention in the CNN documentary *Weed.*[25] Often these young patients need a higher amount of CBD to reach their therapeutic goals. Recently a pharmaceutical-grade CBD has been approved by the FDA. It is called Epidiolex and is a CBD isolate, which is to say it is pure CBD with no THC. The recommended dosing for Epidiolex is 20 mg/kg, an extremely high dose. A child weighing 40 pounds, for example, would receive about 360 mg of CBD every day. But cannabis physicians using full-spectrum CBD, often derived from high-grade hemp, have found that doses as low as 1 to 5 mg/kg can be effective. This means that a 40-pound child would receive about 91 mg a day. And you can see there is lots of room to titrate upward.

Dosage for Multiple Ailments

Many patients will suffer from more than one ailment. In medical parlance this is called comorbidity. A diabetic patient may develop cancer, or an anxiety patient may also have insomnia and perhaps irritable bowel syndrome. It is quite possible that CBD can treat the symptoms of these comorbid ailments, but dosing does become a bit more complex, and patients using CBD in these situations must exercise caution and patience. It is not uncommon for a patient with one ailment, for example cancer, to start using CBD to treat the pain or perhaps the nausea caused by anticancer drugs and then realize that their insomnia has eased or disappeared.

For patients with comorbidities, the best advice is to determine your primary goal in using CBD and record that goal in a CBD journal. Use the journal to keep track of goals, dosing, and results. "Start low and go slow" still applies. Keep in mind that CBD is interacting with your ECS. It can be a delicate process to tune the ECS system, particularly if you have more than one ailment.

Another consideration is the delivery method. For example, a CBD tincture in the evening may help with insomnia while a CBD salve or ointment can help with arthritic pain on an as-needed basis. For a fibromyalgia patient, the routine use of CBD capsules may help relieve pain while a cannabis tincture can be used when anxiety flares. Use common sense and keep in mind the various delivery methods of CBD that are available.

The goal in any cannabinoid regimen is to use as little as possible to achieve the therapeutic effect. Start your therapy at the lowest dose (0.01 mg/kg) or at the dose recommended by your healthcare provider.

In the Less Method chart on page 58, you have a handy reference point to start low and go slow. Start by locating your weight in the left-hand column; the next column converts that weight to kilograms. Then follow across that row to see the proper dosing for five different doses of CBD. For example, if you weigh 130 pounds, your kilogram weight is 59.1 (130 lb. ÷ 2.2 = 59.1 kg). Starting at the lowest dose of 0.01 mg/kg, you multiply that by your kilogram weight: 0.01 × 59.1 = .591 mg of CBD each day. Rounding off is acceptable. In this example it may be easier for you to round off to 0.6 mg/kg. Given in two doses, that would be 0.3 mg in the morning and 0.3 mg in the late afternoon or evening.

CHART 3: The Less Method—
Start Low and Go Slow with CBD Therapy

YOUR WEIGHT IN POUNDS	YOUR WEIGHT IN KILOGRAMS	DOSE IS 0.01 MG/KG A DAY, THEN TOTAL DOSE IS . . .	DOSE IS 0.03 MG/KG A DAY, THEN TOTAL DOSE IS . . .
70	31.8	0.32	0.95
80	36.4	0.36	1.09
90	40.9	0.41	1.23
100	45.5	0.45	1.36
110	50.0	0.50	1.50
120	54.5	0.55	1.64
130	59.1	0.59	1.77
140	63.6	0.64	1.91
150	68.2	0.68	2.05
160	72.7	0.73	2.18
170	77.3	0.77	2.32
180	81.8	0.82	2.45
190	86.4	0.86	2.59
200	90.9	0.91	2.73
210	95.5	0.95	2.86
220	100.0	1.00	3.00
230	104.5	1.05	3.14
240	109.1	1.09	3.27
250	113.6	1.14	3.41
260	118.2	1.18	3.55
270	122.7	1.23	3.68
280	127.3	1.27	3.82
290	131.8	1.32	3.95
300	136.4	1.36	4.09

DOSE IS 0.05 MG/KG A DAY, THEN TOTAL DOSE IS ...	DOSE IS 0.075 MG/KG A DAY, THEN TOTAL DOSE IS ...	DOSE IS 0.10 MG/KG A DAY, THEN TOTAL DOSE IS ...
1.59	2.39	3.18
1.82	2.73	3.64
2.05	3.07	4.09
2.27	3.41	4.55
2.50	3.75	5.00
2.73	4.09	5.45
2.95	4.43	5.91
3.18	4.77	6.36
3.41	5.11	6.82
3.64	5.45	7.27
3.86	5.80	7.73
4.09	6.14	8.18
4.32	6.48	8.64
4.55	6.82	9.09
4.77	7.16	9.55
5.00	7.50	10.00
5.23	7.84	10.45
5.45	8.18	10.91
5.68	8.52	11.36
5.91	8.86	11.82
6.14	9.20	12.27
6.36	9.55	12.73
6.59	9.89	13.18
6.82	10.23	13.64

AILMENTS AND RECOMMENDATIONS

Addiction and Alcoholism

Addiction is a common affliction that can be both physically and mentally painful. The reasons for addiction are voluminous and far beyond the scope of this book. While some may have an interest in why addiction occurs, most are looking for ways to solve the problem rather than for an academic treatise on the causes.

CBD offers the addicted individual a new tool for battling this age-old affliction. Its promise is spectacular. In an extensive 2018 study conducted in the United States, involving animal models (rats), the authors found "CBD produced unexpected long-lasting 'therapeutic' effects following only brief treatment. . . . Further adding to the treatment promise of CBD, the efficacy of the cannabinoid to reduce reinstatement in rats with both alcohol and cocaine—and, as previously reported, heroin—histories predicts therapeutic potential for addiction treatment across several classes of abused drugs."[26]

Another study, also using animal models and published in *Frontiers in Pharmacology*, was equally positive: "Experimental studies find that CBD reduces the overall level of alcohol drinking in animal models of [alcohol use disorder] by reducing ethanol intake, motivation for ethanol, relapse, anxiety, and impulsivity."[27] The authors also concluded that CBD helped retain and repair the health of the liver and reduced alcohol-related brain damage.

On a more real-world basis, researchers have reported that in states with operational medical cannabis laws, opioid prescriptions and opioid deaths have been reduced.[28] That research came under some fire when another study disputed the correlation between legal medical cannabis and reduced opioid consumption, but closer examination of that study revealed the researchers used data from states that had medical cannabis laws but whose medical cannabis programs were not yet operational.

CBD offers a wide range of therapeutic use for the addicted person. It can help reduce intake and appears to help individuals stay away from the addictive substance. The cannabinoid helps reduce anxiety associated with withdrawal and also contributes to some behavior modification by reducing impulsiveness.

Ideal Delivery Method: Different routes of administration will produce different effects. Individuals can choose which option works best for them based on their goals. See chapter 2 for more details on routes of administration. Depending on the severity of the disease, multiple routes of administration may be most effective. Inhalation allows for the quick onset of CBD and may help with intense cravings as the individual comes off of the addictive substances. For longer lasting effects, a tincture, capsule, and transdermal patch may be most suitable to control cravings consistently throughout the day.

CBD Dosage: Determining dosages can be complicated. Always start low and slow. Multiple factors need to be considered when developing a CBD treatment plan. Without double-blind human clinical trials to address CBD dosages for certain conditions, we must rely on preclinical (animal) data. It can be difficult to apply dosages from animal studies to humans, and extreme caution must be used. In an article by Gonzales-Cuevas et al. (2018), CBD dosages in rats ranged from 15 mg/kg to 30 mg/kg.[29] In an average human who weighs about 170 pounds, that would equal 1,155 mg CBD and 2,310 mg CBD. While those dosages are likely to be well tolerated in humans, it is unknown if those amounts are necessary. Lower dosages may be effective at managing symptoms. As always, it is best to start low and slow, record your experience, and work closely with a knowledgeable cannabis healthcare practitioner. Keeping a journal with the dose, time of day, and effects will help the individual find the right dose and frequency for their particular condition.

Precautions: Caution should always be taken when an individual begins a CBD regimen, especially if the individual is taking medications or has a history of chronic illnesses.

Commonly Prescribed Drugs and Potential Drug Interactions: For alcoholism: disulfiram (Antabuse), naltrexone (Revia), acamprosate (Campral), gabapentin (Neurontin), and topiramate (Topamax). For opioid addiction: methadone, buprenorphine (Butrans), naltrexone (Revia). See chart 5 on page 116 for possible CBD interactions.

Alzheimer's Disease (AD)

While we may not normally associate Alzheimer's disease (AD) with physical pain, there can be intense anxiety leading to psychological pain that is frightening for patient and caregiver alike. Similarly, some AD patients can become aggressive, even violent, leading to injury of the patient or caregivers. And all dementia patients are at high risk for falls and other circumstances that can cause pain. Memory loss and confusion are the primary hallmarks of AD as well as problems with communication and disruption of normal sleep cycles.

AD is a complicated disease and not fully understood. But we do know there is significant neural degeneration and synaptic loss. Because CBD has neuroprotective properties, it can be useful in treating Alzheimer's. According to Dementia Care Central, "researchers at California's Salk Institute, [in] their 2017 study have found evidence that cannabinoids such as CBD could help remove dementia from brain cells."[30]

Preliminary research has shown that numerous cannabinoids may be effective in treating AD and other forms of dementia. A 2019 article in *Molecular Neurobiology* concluded that "non-psychoactive cannabinoids are potential lead drug candidates for AD and other neurodegenerative diseases."[31]

Ideal Delivery Method: Different routes of administration will produce different effects. Individuals can choose which option works best for them based on their goals. See chapter 2 for more details on routes of administration. The unpredictable nature of Alzheimer's can make administration of medication difficult. The disease can become so severe that some patients forget how to swallow, which makes oral administration difficult. If the patient can swallow sufficiently, then capsules are recommended, since capsules are familiar to the patient. Tinctures can be useful, but an AD patient may not understand the need to retain the tincture in the mouth for optimum absorption. In other words, exact dosing can be a problem. Transdermal patches could be effective and provide the longest relief, but be certain to protect the patch from prying, forgetful fingers. Vaping is not recommended.

CBD Dosage: Determining dosages can be complicated. Always start low and slow. Multiple factors need to be considered when developing a CBD treatment plan. Without double-blind, human clinical trials to address CBD dosages for certain conditions, we must rely on pre-clinical (animal) data. It can be difficult to apply dosages from animal studies to humans, and extreme caution must be used. Unfortunately, extremely high dosing is needed to unlock CBD's neuroprotective properties. A dose of 10 to 20 mg/kg is required, and in a 150-pound (68 kg) individual this could be in the range of 680 to 1,360 mg of CBD every day. Not only is this expensive, but it can also be hard to find high-dose CBD capsules, meaning the patient may have to take a multitude of capsules. If you are fortunate enough to live in a legal medical cannabis state, it is more economical, and probably more effective, to locate a full-spectrum product with CBD and THC or CBD and CBN. Keeping a journal with the dose, time of day, and effects will help the individual find the right dose and frequency for their particular condition.

While most studies on CBD for Alzheimer's disease focus on using it as a treatment, there are suitable usages of CBD for symptom management. Late-stage Alzheimer's patients may develop extreme anxiety and/or agitation. CBD can be effective at managing those symptoms with little to no side effects. For more information, see Anxiety Disorders on page 66.

Precautions: Caution should always be taken when an individual begins a CBD regimen, especially if the individual is taking medications or has a history of chronic illnesses.

AD presents special challenges because often the patient is unable to communicate. Therefore, a caregiver must be particularly vigilant when administering any cannabinoids. Of course, you should start low and go slow. CBD will not cause a high, but it does have effects (see chapter 1).

Commonly Prescribed Drugs and Potential Drug Interactions: donepezil (Aricept), rivastigmine (Exelon), galantamine (Razadyne), and quetiapine (Seroquel).

Please consult your healthcare practitioner or a knowledgeable cannabis healthcare provider who can review your medications prior to starting cannabis therapy and continue to monitor you during the duration of treatment. Currently, there are no studies specifically addressing CBD and typical AD drugs. See chart 5 on page 116 for possible CBD interactions.

Amyotrophic Lateral Sclerosis (ALS)

Also known as Lou Gehrig's disease, this affects the motor neurons of the spinal cord, causing progressive weakness and muscle atrophy, particularly in the voluntary muscles that allow us to walk, speak, and eat. It is named for a baseball great who died of the disease in

1941. Stephen Hawking, the brilliant physicist, may be the best known contemporary sufferer. ALS patients experience pain, depression, dementia, sleep disorders, and Parkinsonism.

There have been promising studies of cannabinoids in mice with ALS, although it does seem mixtures with THC are more effective than CBD alone. A 2016 study from the *Neural Regeneration Research* journal concluded "there is a valid rationale to propose the use of cannabinoid compounds in the pharmacological management of ALS patients. Cannabinoids indeed are able to delay ALS progression and prolong survival."[32] In Australia there is an ongoing clinical trial with CBD oil and ALS patients that is estimated to continue until January 2021.

Ideal Delivery Method: Different routes of administration will produce different effects. Individuals can choose which option works best for them based on their goals (see chapter 2 for more details on routes of administration). Because ALS affects voluntary muscles, dosing can be difficult, particularly as the disease progresses. It is noteworthy that ALS patients who use cannabis often express the belief that THC is more helpful, and at least one patient prefers to smoke cannabis,[33] claiming the THC helps control her disease and smoking allows for rapid onset of relief. As the disease progresses, it may be difficult for the individual with ALS to use their chest muscles, and inhalation may no longer be an option. Using tinctures, capsules, and/or transdermal patches may be more beneficial for long-term use of CBD.

CBD Dosage: Determining dosages can be complicated. Always start low and go slow. Multiple factors need to be considered when developing a CBD treatment plan. Without double-blind human clinical trials to address CBD dosages for certain conditions, we must rely on preclinical (animal) data. It can be difficult to apply dosages from animal studies to humans, and extreme caution must be used. There is one published case study that provides good direction with respect to CBD dosing, although the patient did eventually switch to THC.[34] This result is in keeping with other patient reports that claim THC is an important component of effective cannabinoid treatment of ALS. Keeping a journal with the dose, time of day, and effects will help the individual find the right dose and frequency for their particular condition.

Precautions: Caution should always be taken when an individual begins a CBD regimen, especially if the individual is taking medications or has a history of chronic illnesses.

Drug purity would be particularly important for ALS patients, since many substances can attack the motor neurons.

Commonly Prescribed Drugs and Potential Drug Interactions: riluzole (Rilutek), dextromethorphan (Tussin), quinidine (Nuedexta), and edaravone (Radicava).

Please consult your healthcare practitioner or a knowledgeable cannabis healthcare provider who can review your medications prior to starting cannabis therapy and continue to monitor you during the duration of treatment. See chart 5 on page 116 for possible CBD interactions.

Anxiety Disorders

Anxiety is a normal emotion that everyone experiences from time to time. Anxiety can be related to events, like public speaking, visiting a doctor, holidays, and family gatherings. Anxiety can also be associated with disease process. Cancer patients, for example, often experience anxiety as a result of their diagnosis and treatments. For these types of temporary anxieties, CBD can be a welcome "take as needed" medication.

But there are other, far more complex and insidious forms of anxiety that can virtually hobble an individual's life, rendering them helpless, isolated, and living in fear. According to the National Institute of Mental Health, an estimated 19 percent of US adults had an anxiety disorder in the past year.[35]

The calming effect of CBD makes it a natural for treatment of anxiety. In some regards treating anxiety is CBD's main function, since the cannabinoid serves as a natural modifier for THC, its psychoactive cannabinoid companion.

A recent study published in *The Permanente Journal* (January 2019) concluded "CBD appears to be better tolerated than routine psychiatric medications. Furthermore, CBD displays promise as a tool for reducing anxiety in clinical populations."[36]

Ideal Delivery Method: Different routes of administration will produce different effects. Individuals can choose which option works best for them based on their goals. See chapter 2 for more details on routes of administration. For more immediate relief, CBD can be inhaled (vaped), and patients can experience potential relief within minutes. This route of administration may be best for those who suffer from panic attacks or extreme anxiety. Using an oral preparation or a transdermal patch of CBD is best for longer-lasting relief of anxiety and may be used in conjunction with inhalation. Depending on the severity of the anxiety, multiple routes of administration may be necessary to control symptoms throughout the day. Topicals are not appropriate, as they will not provide systemic relief and are very unpredictable with respect to onset.

CBD Dosage: Determining dosages can be complicated. Always start low and go slow. Multiple factors need to be considered when developing a CBD treatment plan. Without double-blind human clinical trials to address CBD dosages for certain conditions, we must rely on preclinical (animal) data. It can be difficult to apply dosages from animal studies to humans, and extreme caution must be used. Additionally, CBD can have a bidirectional effect. Small doses may be stimulating, like caffeine. In those dosages, CBD may exacerbate anxiety. Large dosages may be more calming and/or relaxing. In a recent study out of Colorado, researchers found that a 25 mg capsule of CBD daily reduced anxiety significantly.[37] Keeping a journal with the dose, time of day, and effects will help the individual find the right dose and frequency for their particular condition.

Precautions: Caution should always be taken when an individual begins a CBD regimen, especially if the individual is taking medications or has a history of chronic illnesses. CBD can have biphasic properties, meaning that a low dose may have one effect and a higher dose may have the opposite effect. Some patients have reported that low doses of CBD increased anxiety.

Commonly Prescribed Drugs and Potential Drug Interactions: alprazolam (Xanax), lorazepam (Ativan), clonazepam (Klonopin), and diazepam (Valium); citalopram (Celexa), escitalopram (Lexapro), fluoxetine (Prozac), paroxetine (Paxil), sertraline (Zoloft), and venlafaxine (Effexor); duloxetine (Cymbalta); gabapentin (Neurontin) and pregabalin (Lyrica); propranolol (Inderal); hydroxyzine (Atarax); and buspirone (BuSpar).

Medication classes such as antidepressants, antihistamines, beta-blockers, anticonvulsants, benzodiazepines, and antianxiety drugs are recommended in the treatment of generalized anxiety disorder and panic attacks. Antidepressants, particularly SSRIs (selective serotonin reuptake inhibitors), can be helpful for chronic anxiety. Antihistamines and beta-blockers are more commonly used for social or performance anxiety. The use of anticonvulsants for anxiety is a more recent discovery and has shown some promise in the treatment of chronic anxiety. Benzodiazepines are more commonly used for panic attacks.

Please consult your healthcare practitioner or a knowledgeable cannabis healthcare provider who can review your medications prior to starting cannabis therapy and continue to monitor you during the duration of treatment. See chart 5 on page 116 for possible CBD interactions.

Arthritis

According to the Arthritis Foundation, 54 million Americans currently have arthritis, and by 2040 that number is likely to increase to 78 million. Like cancer, arthritis is not just one disease but more than 100 different conditions collected under the umbrella title of "arthritis." Regardless of the type of arthritis, there is pain associated with the disease that can range from moderate to severe. The most common is osteoarthritis (OA), afflicting more than 21 million Americans. OA attacks the joints, causing inflammation and pain. This can lead to degeneration of the cartilage and become disabling.

Rheumatoid arthritis (RA), an autoimmune disorder, primarily attacks the body's joints but can also affect body systems such as the cardiovascular or respiratory systems. About 1.5 million Americans suffer from RA. It is a painful, progressive disease that often requires biological agents to modify and manage the condition.

The Arthritis Foundation has been carefully monitoring the growing CBD market, particularly among their constituents. In July 2019 they conducted a survey of 2,600 arthritis patients and discovered that nearly 80 percent are currently using CBD, have used it in the past, or are considering using it. This led the foundation to compile "CBD Guidance for Adults with Arthritis."[38]

A 2019 German study took advantage of legal access to Sativex, the THC:CBD oral mucosa spray from GW Pharmaceutical, and conducted a real-world study of 800 chronic pain patients. The study concluded that "THC:CBD oromucosal spray proved to be an effective and well-tolerated add-on treatment for patients with elsewhere refractory chronic pain—especially of neuropathic origin."[39]

Recent research involving transdermal application of CBD on arthritic rats was also very encouraging, showing "significantly reduced joint swelling, limb posture scores as a rating of spontaneous pain, immune cell infiltration and thickening of the synovial membrane in a dose-dependent manner."[40]

Ideal Delivery Method: Different routes of administration will produce different effects. Individuals can choose which option works best for them based on their goals. See chapter 2 for more details on routes of administration. Depending on the severity of the disease, multiple routes of administration may be most effective. Topical preparations of CBD such as lotions or salves are ideal for those with less severe arthritis. The patient can apply the topical directly to the affected area. For advanced arthritis patients with multiple sites of inflammation, a more systemic approach may be desirable, such as capsules or a tincture. Transdermal patches can also be effective systemically. RA may benefit more from the systemic anti-inflammatory benefits of tinctures and/or capsules.

CBD Dosage: Determining dosages can be complicated. Always start low and go slow. Multiple factors need to be considered when developing a CBD treatment plan. Without double-blind human clinical trials to address CBD dosages for certain conditions, we must rely on preclinical (animal) data. It can be difficult to apply dosages from animal studies to humans, and extreme caution must be used. The Arthritis Foundation website[41] is extremely helpful for the patient seeking information on CBD. The website also contains dosing recommendations from a physician that suggests "5–10 mg twice daily, and then slowly increase, going up to a dose of 50–100 mg per day. If that doesn't help, try a CBD product with a low dose of THC."

Precautions: Caution should always be taken when an individual begins a CBD regimen, especially if the individual is taking medications or has a history of chronic illnesses.

Commonly Prescribed Drugs and Potential Drug Interactions: aspirin (Bayer), naproxen (Aleve), ibuprofen (Advil), celecoxib (Celebrex), hydrocodone or oxycodone (Vicodin or Roxicodone), adalimumab (Humira), methotrexate (Trexall), prednisone (Deltasone), and etanercept (Enbrel).

There are numerous drugs used in the treatment of arthritis. This is just a partial list. Please consult your healthcare practitioner or a knowledgeable cannabis healthcare provider who can review your medications prior to starting cannabis therapy and continue to monitor you during the duration of treatment. See chart 5 on page 116 for possible CBD interactions.

Cancer

Cancer comes in many forms, and CBD's role in the treatment of cancer depends on many variables. Entire books have been and will be written on this topic. This book is focused on pain relief using CBD, but patients should also be aware that research has shown cannabinoids have antitumor properties in animal studies and there have been many anecdotal accounts of cured cancers after using cannabinoids. A recent survey found that only 15 percent of cancer patients received information on cannabis from their care team.[42] Cancer patients are looking to CBD for symptom relief, and many of them are turning to the Internet for answers. For a trusted and in-depth discussion of cannabinoids and cancer therapy, please visit Project CBD online.

Cancer and the treatment associated with it can produce many symptoms. CBD may be useful in treating the side effects related to chemotherapy such as nausea and vomiting, appetite loss, insomnia, anxiety, depression, fatigue, and peripheral neuropathy. Additionally, cancer patients may experience pain from the cancer itself or from the treatment, and CBD has shown promise in reducing opioid use when administered simultaneously.

CBD may offer patients the ability to control their symptoms without needing multiple different medications, thereby reducing their overall intake of pharmaceuticals and eliminating additional side effects from other medications.

Multiple animal studies have demonstrated that CBD can decrease nausea and vomiting related to chemotherapy. Low dosages were more effective, whereas higher dosages did not help chemotherapy-induced nausea and vomiting.[43]

Ideal Delivery Method: Different routes of administration will produce different effects. Individuals can choose which option works best for them based on their goals. See chapter 2 for more details on routes of administration. Depending on the severity of the disease, multiple routes of administration may be most effective.

CBD Dosage: Determining dosages can be complicated. Always start low and go slow. Multiple factors need to be considered when developing a CBD treatment plan. Without double-blind human clinical trials to address CBD dosages for certain conditions, we must rely on preclinical (animal) data. It can be difficult to apply dosages from animal studies to humans, and extreme caution must be used.

Precautions: Caution should always be taken when an individual begins a CBD regimen, especially if the individual is taking medications or has a history of chronic illnesses. Cancer patients who are undergoing chemotherapy or who are known to be immunocompromised must obtain products that have gone through rigorous testing for molds, fungus, heavy metals, and pesticides to ensure that there are no harmful contaminants. Because CBD can often impact the levels of other medications, taking it with oral chemotherapy/biotherapy medications may influence the levels of the medications and/or the CBD. It is imperative that patients who are taking oral medications specifically to treat their cancer have a medical professional do a thorough medication review to identify possible interactions and reduce side effects.

Commonly Prescribed Drugs and Potential Drug Interactions: ondansetron (Zofran), granisetron (Sustol), palonosetron (Aloxi), aprepitant (Emend), dexamethasone (DexPak), duloxetine (Cymbalta), prednisone (Deltasone), gabapentin (Neurontin) and pregabalin (Lyrica), dronabinol (Marinol), nabilone (Cesamet), hydrocodone (Vicodin), oxycodone (Roxicodone), alprazolam (Xanax), lorazepam (Ativan), clonazepam (Klonopin) and diazepam (Valium), citalopram (Celexa), escitalopram (Lexapro), eluxadoline (Viberzi), paroxetine (Paxil), sertraline (Zoloft), venlafaxine (Effexor), trazodone (Desyrel), zolpidem (Ambien), temazepam (Restoril), and eszopiclone (Lunesta).

This is a list of drugs commonly prescribed to cancer patients. It is by no means complete. Please consult your healthcare practitioner or a knowledgeable cannabis healthcare provider who can review your medications prior to starting cannabis therapy and continue to monitor you during the duration of treatment. See chart 5 on page 116 for possible CBD interactions.

Currently, there are two FDA-approved synthetic THC cannabinoid products available by prescription: dronabinol and nabilone. Both are primarily used to treat the nausea, vomiting, and appetite loss associated with chemotherapy treatments. Other treatments for symptom management include anti-nausea medications, steroids, appetite stimulants, anticonvulsants, pain medications, antidepressants, antianxiety medications, and sleep aids. Some patients may be prescribed oral medications to treat the cancer itself. Those may include chemotherapy, biotherapy, and/or hormone blocking pills.

Chronic Pain

George Orwell captured the essence of chronic pain when he wrote, "Of pain you could wish only one thing: that it should stop."[44]

Statistics suggest there are literally millions of Americans who understand and agree with Mr. Orwell's assessment. A 2011 report from the Institute of Medicine states that 40 percent of Americans, approximately 100 million people, live with chronic pain. While some of that pain may be caused by the specific ailments listed in this book, there are many individuals who are suffering chronic pain as the result of accidents, poor working or environmental conditions, orthopedic deterioration from sports, or simply living. For these individuals, CBD offers a new tool in their constant battle against chronic pain.

Chronic pain usually begins with an initial injury—examples include a pulled muscle or sprain, a broken bone, and a car accident with resulting injury—that leads to inflammation and nerve damage. Even after the initial injury heals, the pain lingers. If it lingers beyond 12 weeks, it is considered to be chronic pain.

The goal in treating chronic pain is to ease the pain without compromising a patient's activity level, mental functions, or emotional health. Over-the-counter (OTC) drugs such as acetaminophen and ibuprofen can do the job of relieving pain for some patients, but many patients are moved onto opioid drugs when OTC drugs fail. This happens even though there is no evidence to support the benefit of opioids in chronic pain treatment. In fact, in 2015 the *Annals of Internal Medicine* published a study that confirmed "evidence is insufficient to determine the effectiveness of long-term opioid therapy for improving chronic pain and function." With the changes in opioid prescribing practices, other medications like antidepressants and anticonvulsants may be used to control pain.

All of this has made CBD a particularly welcome addition to the medical regime of chronic pain sufferers. CBD's ability to reduce inflammation and serve as a neuroprotectant makes it very appropriate for pain relief. A 2016 study conducted in Michigan, a medical cannabis state, found that 64 percent of medical cannabis users reported reduced opioid use. And there was more. The researchers wrote, "This study suggests that many chronic pain (CP) patients are essentially substituting medical cannabis for opioids and other medications for CP treatment, and finding the benefit and side effect profile of cannabis to be greater than these other classes of medications."[45]

Ideal Delivery Method: Different routes of administration will produce different effects. Individuals can choose which option works best for them based on their goals. See chapter 2 for more details on routes of administration. Depending on the severity of the disease, multiple routes of administration may be most effective. Because chronic pain comes in so many variations, there is no one ideal delivery method. Many patients will benefit from multiple different routes of administration. In some cases, inhalation may provide immediate relief for intense breakthrough pain whereas tinctures, capsules, topicals, or transdermal patches may provide longer-lasting relief. If pain is localized, a patient may find topical preparations work well enough. Edibles can be erratic in dosing and are not recommended for a new user.

CBD Dosages: Determining dosages can be complicated. Always start low and go slow. Multiple factors need to be considered when developing a CBD treatment plan. Without double-blind human clinical trials to address CBD dosages for certain conditions, we must rely on preclinical (animal) data. It can be difficult to apply dosages from animal studies to humans, and extreme caution must be used. Many patients have found that using CBD with opioids reduces their overall opioid intake and shifts the dysphoria associated with chronic pain.[46]

Precautions: Caution should always be taken when an individual begins a CBD regimen, especially if the individual is taking medications or has a history of chronic illnesses. Patients who are using CBD and opioids need to work closely with their healthcare practitioner, especially if they choose to wean down or off opioids.

Commonly Prescribed Drugs and Potential Drug Interactions: aspirin (Bayer), naproxen (Aleve), ibuprofen (Advil), fentanyl (Duragesic), celecoxib (Celebrex), hydrocodone (Vicodin), oxycodone (Roxicodone), duloxetine (Cymbalta), gabapentin (Neurontin), pregabalin (Lyrica), tramadol (Ultram), and methadone.

This is a not a complete list of medications. Please consult your health-care practitioner or a knowledgeable cannabis healthcare provider who can review your medications prior to starting cannabis therapy and continue to monitor you during the duration of treatment. See chart 5 on page 116 for possible CBD interactions.

Diabetic Peripheral Neuropathy/General Neuropathy

Neuropathic pain accompanies many ailments but may be more common among individuals with diabetes or those who have received certain chemotherapy agents or from excessive alcohol intake.

The discovery of the endocannabinoid system (see chapter 1) and the realization of its important role in homeostasis opened an ever-expanding landscape of possible therapeutic applications for cannabis. Its effectiveness as a pain medication is often cited in historical documents, and upon discovery of the neuroprotective role of cannabinoids, scientists were quick to put together the pieces, realizing that cannabinoids could have a profound effect on a multitude of illnesses.

As early as 2003, articles about cannabinoids and neuropathic pain were appearing with comments such as "data supports the interest in the evaluation of cannabinoids as an alternative for the treatment of neuropathic pain and the involvement of the endocannabinoid system in the modulation of neuropathic pain perception is being widely studied."[47]

Today, there are numerous studies underway exploring the use of cannabinoids in treating not only diabetic peripheral neuropathy but possibly diabetes in general. Diabetes.co.uk wrote in its newsletter, "Chronic inflammation has long been known to play a key role in the development of insulin resistance and therefore type 2 diabetes.

[Cannabis] researchers believe that the anti-inflammatory properties of CBD could treat this inflammation and therefore improve the body's metabolism."[48]

Additionally, CBD is showing promise in chemotherapy-induced peripheral neuropathy. In one animal study, researchers found that administering CBD 30 minutes prior to Paclitaxel significantly reduced and, in some mice, prevented chemotherapy-induced peripheral neuropathy without compromising the antitumor effects of the chemotherapy.[49]

Ideal Delivery Method: Different routes of administration will produce different effects. Individuals can choose which option works best for them based on their goals. See chapter 2 for more details on routes of administration. Depending on the severity of the disease, multiple routes of administration may be most effective. Capsules or tinctures would be best for continuing therapy, but salves and ointments can provide relief during flare-ups.

CBD Dosage: Determining dosages can be complicated. Always start low and go slow. Multiple factors need to be considered when developing a CBD treatment plan. Without double-blind human clinical trials to address CBD dosages for certain conditions, we must rely on preclinical (animal) data. It can be difficult to apply dosages from animal studies to humans, and extreme caution must be used. A study using Sativex, a THC and CBD oral spray with 2.7 mg THC and 2.5 mg CBD, found that peripheral neuropathy pain was reduced by 30 percent compared to the group that did not receive Sativex.[50]

Precautions: Caution should always be taken when an individual begins a CBD regimen, especially if the individual is taking medications or has a history of chronic illnesses. Since CBD can cause dizziness, it is important to evaluate for balance issues associated with peripheral neuropathy to avoid any unwanted falls.

Commonly Prescribed Drugs and Potential Drug Interactions: dulox-etine (Cymbalta), gabapentin (Neurontin), pregabalin (Lyrica), venlafaxine (Effexor), tramadol (Ultram), amitriptyline (Elavil), nortrip-tyline (Pamelor), oxcarbazepine (Oxtellar), and capsaicin.

A recent study of commonly prescribed medications for diabetic neu-ropathy was reviewed in March 2017 at WebMD. "In the new study, the Hopkins group reviewed 106 studies on pain relief for diabetic neuropathy. The researchers found 'moderate' evidence that the anti-depressants duloxetine (Cymbalta) and venlafaxine (Effexor) reduce diabetic nerve pain. However, they only found 'weak' evidence that botulinum toxin (Botox), the anti-seizure drugs pregabalin (Lyrica) and oxcarbazepine (Trileptal), and drugs called tricyclic antidepressants and atypical opioids (drugs such as Tramadol) may help reduce pain."[51] Opioid use has not proven to be effective for neuropathic pain and is best avoided.

Please consult your healthcare practitioner or a knowledgeable can-nabis healthcare provider who can review your medications prior to starting cannabis therapy and continue to monitor you during the duration of treatment. See chart 5 on page 116 for possible CBD interactions.

Fibromyalgia (FM)

Fibromyalgia (FM) is characterized by widespread pain, a heightened pain response to pressure, extreme fatigue, sleep problems, and some cognitive issues, primarily with memory. Its cause is unknown, but there is speculation that both environmental and genetic factors may be at play. In the last decade, Dr. Ethan Russo has also theorized that FM may be related to a dysfunctional endogenous cannabinoid system.

For many years, there was controversy about FM and whether it was truly a disease or a psychological condition, but today it is recog-nized by the National Institutes of Health and the American College of

Rheumatology as a genuine disorder. There is no specific test for FM. Diagnosing the disease consists of ruling out other possible causes for the patient's complaints.

There is substantial interest in the use of CBD for treatment of FM, but the studies to date have been disappointing with respect to the use of only CBD in treating FM. A study published in April 2019 concluded that "a cannabis variety with a high CBD content was devoid of analgesic activity in any of the spontaneous or evoked pain models."[52] This same study, however, reported positive results using THC and THC/CBD tinctures.

This study was small—only 20 patients—and is by no means definitive. There are many anecdotal reports of successful use of CBD in treating the symptoms of FM, and most states with legal medical cannabis programs allow the plant's use for patients with FM. Since CBD contributes to an overall sense of well-being, it could be that this is the effect FM patients are experiencing. Nevertheless, it is clear that cannabis has a future in FM treatments.

Ideal Delivery Method: Different routes of administration will produce different effects. Individuals can choose which option works best for them based on their goals. See chapter 2 for more details on routes of administration. Depending on the severity of the disease, multiple routes of administration may be most effective. Capsules or tinctures can be used together with transdermal patches to offer effective ways of maintaining a therapeutic load. As with chronic pain, fibromyalgia may require multiple methods of administration throughout the day. Oral administration will provide longer lasting relief, and inhalation and topicals may provide some relief for breakthrough pain.

CBD Dosage: Determining dosages can be complicated. Always start low and go slow. Multiple factors need to be considered when developing a CBD treatment plan. Without double-blind human clinical trials to address CBD dosages for certain conditions, we must rely on preclinical (animal) data. It can be difficult to apply dosages from animal studies to humans, and extreme caution must be used. In a small sample of 12 females who had chronic pain as a result of headaches, fibromyalgia, arthralgia, and myalgia, dosages of 150 mg CBD per day significantly reduced pain.[53]

Precautions: Caution should always be taken when an individual begins a CBD regimen, especially if the individual is taking medications or has a history of chronic illnesses.

Commonly Prescribed Drugs and Potential Drug Interactions: According to the Arthritis Foundation, there are several classes of drugs that are commonly used in treating fibromyalgia. They are gabapentinoids, sedatives, serotonin norepinephrine reuptake inhibitors (SNRIs), selective serotonin reuptake inhibitors (SSRIs), and tricyclic compounds. Common drugs include milnacipran (Savella), cyclobenzaprine (Amrix), duloxetine (Cymbalta), gabapentin (Neurontin), pregabalin (Lyrica), venlafaxine (Effexor), tramadol (Ultram), and meloxicam (Vivlodex).

Please consult your healthcare practitioner or a knowledgeable cannabis healthcare provider who can review your medications prior to starting cannabis therapy and continue to monitor you during the duration of treatment. See chart 5 on page 116 for possible CBD interactions.

HIV/AIDS

There was a time when a diagnosis of HIV—human immunodeficiency virus—was a death sentence. In the 1980s there were few medications to treat the virus that becomes AIDS (acquired immune deficiency syndrome). Those that did exist, such as AZT, had horrific side effects like unrelenting nausea and vomiting. AIDS patients learned quickly that smoked cannabis could help stop the nausea and vomiting and also worked as an appetite stimulant.

Today, things are significantly better for persons with HIV/AIDS. Many are now living for decades with the disease, and cannabis is playing a part in this for many patients. Marinol, the legal, synthetic delta-9 THC, is often prescribed for emesis and appetite stimulation. Most states with medical cannabis laws include HIV/AIDS on their list of ailments for which cannabis can be recommended. According to Americans for Safe Access, "The effectiveness of cannabis for treating symptoms related to HIV/AIDS . . . has been recognized by several comprehensive, government-sponsored reviews, including those conducted by the Institute of Medicine (IOM), the U.K. House of Lords Science and Technology Committee, the Australian National Task Force on Cannabis, and others."[54]

The majority of research with cannabis and HIV/AIDS has been focused on THC. For those with HIV/AIDS, it is worthwhile to expand your research beyond this book in order to appreciate the full spectrum of how cannabis can help. Like any virus, HIV causes inflammation of the body's cells, and research has shown that CBD can definitely reduce systemic inflammation while also establishing a sense of well-being and calmness. Supporting this, a study from 2012 found that CBD inhibits growth of tumors in Kaposi sarcoma (KS) patients.[55] This is vitally important, as KS is often seen in late-stage AIDS patients.

Ideal Delivery Method: Different routes of administration will produce different effects. Individuals can choose which option works best for them based on their goals. See chapter 2 for more details on routes of administration. Depending on the severity of the disease, multiple routes of administration may be most effective. Given the wide array of symptoms the HIV/AIDS patient will face, the ideal delivery method is going to vary. Systemic methods such as capsules and tinctures can be used for body aches or appetite stimulation. Topical preparations can be used for aching joints, skin eruptions, or nausea and vomiting. Cautious use of edibles may be appropriate to increase stamina and a sense of well-being.

CBD Dosage: Determining dosages can be complicated. Always start low and go slow. Multiple factors need to be considered when developing a CBD treatment plan. Without double-blind human clinical trials to address CBD dosages for certain conditions, we must rely on preclinical (animal) data. It can be difficult to apply dosages from animal studies to humans, and extreme caution must be used. To date, there are no studies that demonstrate CBD dosages for HIV/AIDs as a treatment. Most patients are using CBD for symptom management. Titrate up slowly, and use the minimal amount of CBD that can give relief from HIV/AIDs symptoms.

Precautions: Caution should always be taken when an individual begins a CBD regimen, especially if the individual is taking medications or has a history of chronic illnesses.

Commonly Prescribed Drugs and Potential Drug Interactions: HIV/ AIDS patients may require a larger number of various medications because the disease is attacking the body's only way of fighting off viruses—the immune system. In fact, the disease can make adjustments to medications used to fight it and actually find a way to render a once effective medication ineffective. One online site[56] lists 50 medications that are available to treat HIV/AIDS. The effects of these powerful drugs can be as devastating as the disease itself, thus requiring even more drugs. Common side effects include diarrhea, dizziness, headaches, fatigue, fever, muscle aches, nausea, and vomiting. CBD can be effective in treating most or all of these side effects, so if you are unable to access medical cannabis, CBD may be helpful.

Most HIV/AIDs drugs are multi-class/combination drugs. Examples include abacavir/dolutegravir/lamivudine (Triumeq), dolutegravir/ rilpivirine (Juluca), elvitegravir/cobicistat/emtricitabine/tenofovir (Stribild), elvitegravir/cobicistat/emtricitabine/tenofovir alafenamide (Genvoya), efavirenz/emtricitabine/tenofovir (Atripla), emtricitabine/ rilpivirine/tenofovir alafenamide (Odefsey), emtricitabine/rilpivirine/

tenofovir disoproxil fumarate (Complera), and bictegravir/emtricit-abine/tenofovir alafenamide (Biktarvy).

Please consult your healthcare practitioner or a knowledgeable can-nabis healthcare provider who can review your medications prior to starting cannabis therapy and continue to monitor you during the duration of treatment. See chart 5 on page 116 for possible CBD interactions.

Huntington's Disease (HD)

Huntington's disease (HD) is a particularly rare genetic disorder affecting fewer than 30,000 people in the United States. It attacks nerve cells in the brain, setting up a devastating process wherein the afflicted individuals lose coordination, cognition deteriorates, there are significant changes in personality, and the patient eventually requires full-time care because he or she is unable to swallow food on his or her own. It almost exclusively affects Western cultures. In Japan it is exceedingly rare, and it is virtually nonexistent in Africa.

There is no cure for HD, and there are very few drugs available to treat symptoms. Treatment is often focused on various therapies such as physical and speech.

With the acknowledged neuroprotective properties of cannabi-noids, it was only natural that researchers would consider using CBD in the treatment of HD. Since the disease is genetic and will occur in 50 percent of children who have a parent with the mutated gene called huntingtin, it is desirable to have some therapy that will help prevent neurodegeneration before it begins.

As early as 1991, researchers were looking at this question and initially concluded cannabinoids were not helpful in treating HD.[57] Ironically, these researchers may have employed too high a dose, administering 700 mg a day of CBD to half of 15 patients (the others received 700 mg of sesame oil). Today, it is understood that less is more, and, as with all other ailments, patients are encouraged to start low and go slow. A study from 2011 found that Sativex, the 1:1 oral spray made by GW Pharmaceuticals, found success with HD patients, and the results were "in support of a beneficial effect of the cannabis-based medicine Sativex as a neuroprotective agent capable of delaying disease progression in HD."[58] However, Sativex is not yet available in the United States.

Depending on the health of the patient's endocannabinoid system, microdosing CBD may be sufficient, with gradual increases as a patient's symptoms dictate (see the Less Method chart in chapter 2).

Ideal Delivery Method: Different routes of administration will produce different effects. Individuals can choose which option works best for them based on their goals. See chapter 2 for more details on routes of administration. Depending on the severity of the disease, multiple routes of administration may be most effective. Initially, if the patient can manage, tinctures may be preferable to allow microdosing. As the need for CBD increases, the patient may move to capsules. Vaping may be effective although difficult as the disease becomes more advanced.

CBD Dosage: Determining dosages can be complicated. Always start low and go slow. Multiple factors need to be considered when developing a CBD treatment plan. Without double-blind human clinical trials to address CBD dosages for certain conditions, we must rely on preclinical (animal) data. It can be difficult to apply dosages from animal studies to humans, and extreme caution must be used. As previously mentioned, HD patients should start with microdosing to determine the efficacy of CBD. Titrate up slowly, and use the minimal amount of CBD that can give relief from HD symptoms.

Precautions: Caution should always be taken when an individual begins a CBD regimen, especially if the individual is taking medications or has a history of chronic illnesses.

In advanced cases it is particularly important to observe for signs of choking while administering any medications.

Commonly Prescribed Drugs and Potential Drug Interactions: Medications prescribed for Huntington's patients fall into two categories: medications for movement disorders and medications for psychiatric disorders. To date, the FDA has not approved any medications to treat the disease. HD patients must rely on medications to control the symptoms of the disease. Common drugs include tetrabenazine (Xenazine), haloperidol (Haldol), quetiapine (Seroquel), risperidone (Risperdal), olanzapine (Zyprexa), and levetiracetam (Keppra).

Please consult your healthcare practitioner or a knowledgeable cannabis healthcare provider who can review your medications prior to starting cannabis therapy and continue to monitor you during the duration of treatment. See chart 5 on page 116 for possible CBD interactions.

Inflammatory Bowel Disease (IBD)

Inflammatory bowel disease (IBD) is an umbrella term for disorders that involve chronic inflammation of the digestive tract. There are two main types: Crohn's disease and ulcerative colitis. The two are different but share common symptoms: diarrhea, abdominal pain and cramping, constipation, fever, reduced appetite, fatigue, blood in stool, and unintended weight loss. The condition afflicts as many as one million Americans and can occur at any age and in any ethnic group.

The two disorders differ in their locales. Crohn's disease causes inflammation throughout the digestive tract whereas ulcerative colitis is situated in the large intestines and rectum, causing large sores in the innermost lining of the colon. Crohn's disease can be far more debilitating, with the inflammation occurring anywhere from the mouth to the anus and affecting both the large and small intestines. The inflammation in Crohn's disease can extend through all layers of the intestine and can affect internal organs.

The benefit of cannabinoids in treating these disorders has been reported anecdotally for years, but now those reports are gaining support from a recent study in England that involved CBD and an endocannabinoid called palmitoylethanolamide (PEA).[59] The researchers in this study concluded that CBD with PEA reduced the permeability of the intestines, allowing the bowels to process foods into the body while blocking harmful bacteria and other substances. This conclusion is of great importance, as it is this permeability that goes haywire in Crohn's and ulcerative colitis.

Another recent study was conducted in Colorado.[60] Surveys were given to IBD patients between the ages of 13 and 23 years. Of the 82 participants, 15 were using cannabis and reported improvement in sleep quality and nausea and an increase in appetite. Six of the 15 used only cannabis oil, and 5 of the 6 described their use as "medical." For these individuals, relieving pain was their primary reason for using cannabis.

Ideal Delivery Method: Different routes of administration will produce different effects. Individuals can choose which option works best for them based on their goals. See chapter 2 for more details on routes of administration. Depending on the severity of the disease, multiple routes of administration may be most effective. Systemic CBD, either through capsules or tinctures, is appropriate. Transdermal patches may be effective and preferable to oral routes of administration.

CBD Dosage: Determining dosages can be complicated. Always start low and go slow. Multiple factors need to be considered when developing a CBD treatment plan. Without double-blind human clinical trials to address CBD dosages for certain conditions, we must rely on preclinical (animal) data. It can be difficult to apply dosages from animal studies to humans, and extreme caution must be used. To date, there are no studies that demonstrate CBD dosages for IBD as a treatment. Most patients are using CBD for symptom management. Titrate up slowly, and use the minimal amount of CBD that can give relief from IBD symptoms.

Precautions: Caution should always be taken when an individual begins a CBD regimen, especially if the individual is taking medications or has a history of chronic illnesses.

Commonly Prescribed Drugs and Potential Drug Interactions: Medications for inflammatory bowel disease fall into three categories: anti-inflammatory, immune system suppressors, and antibiotics. Common drugs include azathioprine (Azasan), mercaptopurine (Purixan), cyclosporine (Restasis), methotrexate (Trexall), infliximab (Remicade), and adalimumab (Humira).

Please consult your healthcare practitioner or a knowledgeable cannabis healthcare provider who can review your medications prior to starting cannabis therapy and continue to monitor you during the duration of treatment. See chart 5 on page 116 for possible CBD interactions.

Irritable Bowel Syndrome (IBS)

It is easy to confuse irritable bowel syndrome (IBS) with inflammatory bowel disease (IBD), but the two are very different. IBS is a functional disorder as opposed to a disease. IBS does not cause inflammation or ulcers. Symptoms include abdominal cramping and pain, gas, bloating, constipation, diarrhea, and mucus in the stool. IBS is sometimes referred to as spastic colon or spastic bowel.[61]

It is estimated that 10 to 15 percent of people in the developed world are affected by IBS, and the condition is more common in South America.[62] Many afflicted with IBS can treat their condition with OTC medications, a change in diet or lifestyle, or a reduction in stress. But others must seek the help of a physician to enable control of their condition.

In 2016, noted cannabis researcher Ethan Russo put forth the theory that conditions such as IBS (as well as migraines, fibromyalgia, and other treatment-resistant syndromes) may be a result of a deficiency in our endocannabinoid systems (see chapter 1 for more on the ECS). With respect to IBS, he noted that the digestive tract is rich with CB2 receptors and hypothesized that "GI propulsion, secretion, and inflammation in the gut are all modulated by the ECS, providing a rationale for cannabinoids as treatment candidates for IBS. As examples, GI propulsion is under tonic control of the ECS, and cannabis was one of the first effective clinical interventions in the 19th century for the intense secretory diarrhea associated with cholera, a finding which was more recently validated with modern methodology."[63]

Specifically, CBD can help with two of the major symptoms of IBS: nausea and abdominal cramping. CBD is tolerated well and has few side effects, especially when compared with some of the side effects of conventional medications.

Ideal Delivery Method: Different routes of administration will produce different effects. Individuals can choose which option works best for them based on their goals. See chapter 2 for more details on routes of administration. Depending on the severity of the disease, multiple routes of administration may be most effective.

CBD Dosage: Determining dosages can be complicated. Always start low and go slow. Multiple factors need to be considered when developing a CBD treatment plan. Without double-blind human clinical trials to address CBD dosages for certain conditions, we must rely on preclinical (animal) data. It can be difficult to apply dosages from animal studies to humans, and extreme caution must be used. To date, there are no studies that demonstrate CBD dosages for IBS as a treatment; however, studies show promise that CBD can reduce inflammation in the gut.[64] Most patients are using CBD for symptom management. Titrate up slowly, and use the minimal amount of CBD that can give relief from IBS symptoms.

Precautions: Caution should always be taken when an individual begins a CBD regimen, especially if the individual is taking medications or has a history of chronic illnesses.

Commonly Prescribed Drugs and Potential Drug Interactions: There are several medications specifically targeting people with IBS. These include alosetron (Lotronex), eluxadoline (Viberzi), rifaximin (Xifaxan), lubiprostone (Amitiza), and linaclotide (Linzess). There are numerous antidiarrheal medications that may be prescribed or recommended. Anticholinergic medication may be prescribed to help with bowel spasms. Tricyclic antidepressants may be prescribed when stress is determined to be a major contributor to IBS.

Please consult your healthcare practitioner or a knowledgeable cannabis healthcare provider who can review your medications prior to starting cannabis therapy and continue to monitor you during the duration of treatment. See chart 5 on page 116 for possible CBD interactions.

Lupus

Lupus is an autoimmune disease that was first recognized in the Middle Ages and has been documented since the mid-1800s. It afflicts 1.5 million Americans and as many as 5 million worldwide. Nine times more women suffer from the disease than men and more women of color than white women.

Lupus has a wide variety of symptoms, which can cause confusion and even delay diagnosis in some cases, but the disease can be diagnosed with a blood test. Symptoms include sensitivity to light, red patches (especially those in the shape of a butterfly), mouth or nose ulcers, arthritis in two or more joints with tenderness or swelling, inflammation of the lining of the heart or lungs, seizures, and excess protein in the urine.

While there are few studies involving CBD and lupus directly, the substantial body of evidence supporting the effectiveness of CBD in treating pain and inflammation would seem to predict its successful use in treating the symptoms of lupus.

According to the Lupus Foundation of America, there is one study underway that is looking at a synthetic derivative of cannabis.[65] The foundation advocates additional research and cautions lupus patients who may be considering treatment with any cannabinoid product to seek the advice of their physician.

Ideal Delivery Method: Different routes of administration will produce different effects. Individuals can choose which option works best for them based on their goals. See chapter 2 for more details on routes of administration. Depending on the severity of the disease, multiple routes of administration may be most effective. Because lupus is a systemic disease, oral medications are usually the best. CBD capsules or tinctures are recommended. Topical salves can be used in cases of joint inflammation. Some lupus patients report relief with transdermal patches, using tinctures as backup.

CBD Dosage: Determining dosages can be complicated. Multiple factors need to be considered when developing a CBD treatment plan. Without double-blind human clinical trials to address CBD dosages for certain conditions, we must rely on preclinical (animal) data. It can be difficult to apply dosages from animal studies to humans, and extreme caution must be used. To date, there are no studies that demonstrate CBD dosages for lupus as a treatment. Most patients are using CBD for symptom management. Titrate up slowly, and use the minimal amount of CBD that can give relief from lupus symptoms.

Precautions: Caution should always be taken when an individual begins a CBD regimen, especially if the individual is taking medications or has a history of chronic illnesses.

Commonly Prescribed Drugs and Potential Drug Interactions:
Autoimmune ailments often call for wide varieties of medications, and lupus is no different. These often include over-the-counter anti-inflammatory medicines such as aspirin and acetaminophen, corticosteroids (for inflammation), antimalarial drugs (for rashes, mouth ulcers, and joint pain), immune modulators (normally used when OTC and corticosteroids fail to reduce inflammation), anti-coagulants, and monoclonal antibodies. Common drugs include hydroxychloroquine (Plaquenil), cyclophosphamide (Cytoxan), azathioprine (Azasan), methotrexate (Trexall), naproxen (Aleve), ibuprofen (Advil), mycophenolate (CellCept), and immune globulin.

Please consult your healthcare practitioner or a knowledgeable can-nabis healthcare provider who can review your medications prior to starting cannabis therapy and continue to monitor you during the dura-tion of treatment. See chart 5 on page 116 for possible CBD interactions.

Lyme Disease

At the beginning of every summer, the warnings are given—cover up, use repellant, and eliminate areas of habitation. It is tick season, and ticks carry Lyme disease. With over 300,000 cases every year in the United States and 65,000 cases in Europe, the warnings are appropri-ate because left untreated, Lyme disease can lead to facial paralysis, joint pain, neck stiffness, and headaches.

Lyme disease is relatively new in terms of medical classification and diagnosis. For decades Lyme disease was misdiagnosed as juvenile rheumatoid arthritis, and it was not until 1975 that the disease was separated from other diagnoses. This event occurred in Old Lyme, Connecticut. In 1981, the bacterium that causes the disease was first described.

The disease is easily diagnosed if caught early and if the telltale red rash with a circular ring is still present. But in some instances that characteristic sign has already faded, and the patient presents with aching muscles, fever, headaches, and swollen lymph nodes—all conditions that could point to dozens of other conditions. There are, however, blood tests that can help rule out other diseases and confirm Lyme disease.

Antibiotic treatment is normally successful, but for a subset of patients the symptoms can linger and sometimes reoccur. It is thought that individuals who have lingering Lyme disease may have autoimmune system issues. It is this category of patients for whom CBD can be most helpful.

CBD does not cure lingering Lyme disease, but it can treat the symptoms, many of which are the same as symptoms from other diseases that benefit from CBD treatment. Joint pain in particular is a potential candidate for CBD. The anti-inflammatory properties of CBD make it a natural to treat this symptom as well as for treatment of swollen lymph nodes. Headaches can also respond to CBD therapy.

Ideal Delivery Method: Different routes of administration will produce different effects. Individuals can choose which option works best for them based on their goals. See chapter 2 for more details on routes of administration. Depending on the severity of the disease, multiple routes of administration may be most effective.

CBD Dosage: Determining dosages can be complicated. Always start low and go slow. Multiple factors need to be considered when developing a CBD treatment plan. Without double-blind human clinical trials to address CBD dosages for certain conditions, we must rely on preclinical (animal) data. It can be difficult to apply dosages from animal studies to humans, and extreme caution must be used. To date, there are no studies that demonstrate CBD dosages for Lyme disease as a treatment. Most patients are using CBD for symptom management. Titrate up slowly, and use the minimal amount of CBD that can give relief from Lyme's symptoms.

Precautions: Caution should always be taken when an individual begins a CBD regimen, especially if the individual is taking medications or has a history of chronic illnesses.

Commonly Prescribed Drugs and Potential Drug Interactions: Oral and intravenous antibiotics are the standard treatment for Lyme disease. Common drugs include doxycycline (Doxy-100), amoxicillin (Moxatag), and cefuroxime (Zinacef).

Please consult your healthcare practitioner or a knowledgeable cannabis healthcare provider who can review your medications prior to starting cannabis therapy and continue to monitor you during the duration of treatment. See chart 5 on page 116 for possible CBD interactions.

Migraines

The Migraine Research Foundation reports that "migraines are an extraordinarily prevalent neurological disease, affecting 39 million men, women, and children in the U.S., and 1 billion worldwide."[66] The severity of migraines is wide ranging, with some lasting for as little as four hours and others continuing for three days.

The underlying cause of migraines is unknown, but there are numerous triggers that are well documented. Stress, anxiety, fatigue, hormonal changes, low blood sugar, and even jet lag are listed as some of the factors that can trigger a migraine.

Specific studies of CBD and migraines are not available, but there is historical data supporting the use of cannabis for headaches.[67] Anecdotal accounts of using cannabis to treat migraines are abundant.

In 2016 a published study in *Pharmacotherapy* documented results from two medical cannabis specialty clinics in Colorado. Between January 2010 and September 2014, 121 patients with a primary diagnosis of migraine headache were recommended medical cannabis as a prophylaxis. Migraine headache frequency decreased from 10.4 to

4.6 headaches per month.[68] This real-world study, with patients using legal cannabis obtained from Colorado dispensaries, may be one of the most helpful studies to migraine sufferers seeking guidance with respect to medical cannabis. The study provides useful data with respect to delivery methods.

In the study, positive effects were reported in 48 patients (39.7 percent), with the most common effects reported being prevention of migraine headache with decreased frequency of migraine headache (24 patients [19.8 percent]) and aborted migraine headache (14 patients [11.6 percent]). Inhaled forms of marijuana were commonly used for acute migraine treatment and were reported to abort migraine headache. Negative effects were reported in 14 patients (11.6 percent); the most common effects were somnolence (2 patients [1.7 percent]) and difficulty controlling the effects of marijuana related to timing and intensity of the dose (2 patients [1.7 percent]), which were experienced only in patients using edible marijuana. Edible marijuana was also reported to cause more negative effects compared with other forms.[69]

It is worth noting that this particular study involved full-spectrum cannabis. It is unclear if CBD alone can provide this level of relief for migraine patients. The ability of CBD to reduce inflammation is certainly beneficial to headache sufferers. In that regard CBD may be most helpful when used at the first signs of a migraine. By reducing inflammation at the start, CBD may lessen the severity and duration of the attack.

Ideal Delivery Method: Different routes of administration will produce different effects. Individuals can choose which option works best for them based on their goals. See chapter 2 for more details on routes of administration. Depending on the severity of the disease, multiple routes of administration may be most effective.

CBD Dosage: Determining dosages can be complicated. Always start low and go slow. Multiple factors need to be considered when developing a CBD treatment plan. Without double-blind human clinical trials to address CBD dosages for certain conditions, we must rely on preclinical (animal) data. It can be difficult to apply dosages from animal studies to humans, and extreme caution must be used. To date, there are no studies that demonstrate CBD dosages for migraines as a treatment. Most patients are using CBD for symptom management, and some have reported dosages between 5 and 50 mg per day are effective at decreasing frequency and intensity of migraines. Titrate up slowly, and use the minimal amount of CBD that can give relief from migraine symptoms.

Precautions: Caution should always be taken when an individual begins a CBD regimen, especially if the individual is taking medications or has a history of chronic illnesses.

Commonly Prescribed Drugs and Potential Drug Interactions: There are several categories of drugs that treat migraines. OTC drugs such as aspirin or ibuprofen may help. Some of these OTC drugs, such as Excedrin Migraine, have a slightly different formulation (added caffeine) that seems to help in cases of mild migraines. Triptans are prescription drugs that block pain pathways to the brain. Examples include sumatriptan and rizatriptan. Dihydroergotamines are available as nasal spray or injection. They are most helpful when taken shortly after the start of a migraine. Patients who cannot take any of the existing migraine medications may find help from opioids, but these are used far less frequently, and only used when other drugs fail.

Please consult your healthcare practitioner or a knowledgeable cannabis healthcare provider who can review your medications prior to starting cannabis therapy and continue to monitor you during the duration of treatment. See chart 5 on page 116 for possible CBD interactions.

Multiple Sclerosis (MS)

Multiple sclerosis (MS) afflicts one million individuals in the United States. It is a disease of the nervous system involving the protective sheath of myelin that surrounds nerves in the brain and spinal cord. This protective sheathing begins to deteriorate, leading to muscle spasticity, double vision, poor concentration, sudden changes in emotion, and loss of bladder control. There is no cure.

The disease can be difficult to diagnose because there is no set pattern of symptoms or deterioration. Further complicating issues is that many patients have spells of remission. In fact, of the four main types of MS—benign, relapse-remitting, secondary progressive, and primary progressive—relapse-remitting is the most common.

Ideal Delivery Method: Different routes of administration will produce different effects. Individuals can choose which option works best for them based on their goals. See chapter 2 for more details on routes of administration. Depending on the severity of the disease, multiple routes of administration may be most effective. MS has the distinction of being the first disease category to have a government-approved cannabis-based medicine developed for it. Sativex (nabiximols) was developed by GW Pharmaceuticals, based in the United Kingdom. Sativex contains almost equal parts of CBD and THC and is an oral mucosa delivery system (i.e., a mouth spray) that delivers a measured dose of 2.5 mg of CBD and 2.7 mg of THC. It was approved in the United Kingdom in 2010 and is now available in 27 countries. The United States is not included among them; however, GW Pharmaceuticals is currently pursuing FDA approval.[70]

CBD Dosing: Determining dosages can be complicated. Always start low and go slow. Multiple factors need to be considered when developing a CBD treatment plan. Without double-blind human clinical trials to address CBD dosages for certain conditions, we must rely on preclinical (animal) data. It can be difficult to apply dosages from animal studies to humans, and extreme caution must be used. The approval of Sativex in the United Kingdom gives MS patients a treasure trove of dosing data on the web. "Start low and go slow" applies to pharmaceutically prepared cannabis-based medicines as well as other brands.[71] GW Pharmaceutical recommends a starting dose of 1 spray with a buildup over two weeks to a maximum of 12 sprays a day (5 in the morning, 7 in the evening). In other words, patients start with a dose of 2.5 mg of CBD and 2.7 mg of THC daily and titrate upwards to a daily dose of 30 mg of CBD and 32.4 mg of THC.[72] These figures can provide goals for those using capsules with the understanding that some of the cannabinoids will be lost in the digestion process.

Precautions: Caution should always be taken when an individual begins a CBD regimen, especially if the individual is taking medications or has a history of chronic illnesses.

Commonly Prescribed Drugs and Potential Drug Interactions: There are very few drugs that are MS-specific. Commonly prescribed drugs fall into several categories: treatments for MS attacks, treatments to modify progression, and treatments for MS signs and symptoms. During an MS attack, corticosteroids will likely be prescribed. To modify progression of the disease, there are numerous drugs: fingolimod (Gilenya), dimethyl fumarate (Tecfidera), teriflunomide (Aubagio), and siponimod (Mayzent). There are several injection and infusion drugs available including ocrelizumab (Ocrevus), glatiramer acetate (Copaxone), natalizumab (Tysabri), beta interferons, alemtuzumab, and mitoxantrone. MS signs and symptoms are treated with a combination of physical therapy, muscle relaxants, medication to reduce fatigue, and increased walking speed. Common drugs include corticosteroids, adrenocorticotrophic hormone (ACTH), immunomodulators (interferon), natalizumab (Tysabri), muscle relaxants such as baclofen (Lioresal) or diazepam (Valium), and carbamazepine (Tegretol). Pain is a particular problem for MS patients because it is often the result of nerve damage, and regular painkillers are ineffective.

Please consult your healthcare practitioner or a knowledgeable cannabis healthcare provider who can review your medications prior to starting cannabis therapy and continue to monitor you during the duration of treatment. See chart 5 on page 116 for possible CBD interactions.

Parkinson's Disease (PD)

Parkinson's disease affects close to one million people in the United States and nearly ten million worldwide, including a number of well-known celebrities: Michael J. Fox, Alan Alda, Linda Ronstadt, and the late Muhammad Ali. Parkinson's disease (PD) can strike both men and women, although men are 1.5 times more likely to be afflicted.

The disease is characterized by involuntary tremors that result from degeneration of the central nervous system. After discovery of the endogenous cannabinoid system (ECS) in the early 1990s, researchers were quick to zero in on the potential of cannabis in treating PD. As one study put it, "The ECS system is emerging as a key regulator of many neuronal systems that are relevant to neurodegenerative disorders."[73]

As with other diseases, CBD can treat multiple symptoms of PD. These include the well-known tremors that are a hallmark of the ailment, but CBD also greatly assists the PD patient with sleep, anxiety, spasticity, reduction of psychotic episodes, and appetite stimulation.

A number of different ailments can have involuntary motor movements that are similar to those seen with Parkinson's disease. These movements, not surprisingly, are called "parkinsonism" and may be responsive to CBD therapy.

Not enough research has been conducted to provide a definitive answer as to how CBD works when combating the symptoms of PD, but the current thinking is that CBD stimulates production of dopamine via the inverse agonist process. A 2017 study discovered "that CBD acts as a novel inverse agonist on both GPR3 and GPR6 indicat[ing] that some of the potential therapeutic effects of CBD (e.g., treatment of Alzheimer's disease and Parkinson's disease) may be mediated through these important receptors."[74] GPR6 helps with the production of dopamine.

Project CBD has a lengthy and thorough discussion of CBD and Parkinson's at www.projectcbd.org/medicine/cbd-and-parkinsons -disease.

Ideal Delivery Method: Different routes of administration will produce different effects. Individuals can choose which option works best for them based on their goals. See chapter 2 for more details on routes of administration. Depending on the severity of the disease, multiple routes of administration may be most effective. Capsules are the optimum delivery method, and high doses may be required.

CBD Dosage: Determining dosages can be complicated. Always start low and go slow. Multiple factors need to be considered when developing a CBD treatment plan. Without double-blind human clinical trials to address CBD dosages for certain conditions, we must rely on preclinical (animal) data. It can be difficult to apply dosages from animal studies to humans, and extreme caution must be used. To date, there are no studies that demonstrate CBD dosages for Parkinson's disease as a treatment. Most patients are using CBD for symptom management, and in one study, 76.9 percent of patients found improved mood, 64 percent found improvement in pain and spasticity, and 59 percent reported decreased tremors and improved quality of sleep.[75] Titrate up slowly, and use the minimal amount of CBD that can give relief from Parkinson's symptoms.

Precautions: Caution should always be taken when an individual begins a CBD regimen, especially if the individual is taking medications or has a history of chronic illnesses.

Commonly Prescribed Drugs and Potential Drug Interactions: Medications used to treat Parkison's disease treat the symptoms, not the actual disease. Most are targeted at treating the tremors and other aspects of motor control. Arriving at the right combination of drugs can be time consuming and frustrating. Drugs include carbidopa-levodopa (Rytary); dopamine agonists such as pramipexole (Mirapex) or ropinirole (Requip); MAO-B inhibitors such as isocarboxazid (Marplan), phenelzine (Nardil), tranylcypromine (Parnate), and selegiline (Eldepryl, Zelapar); catechol O-methyltransferase (COMT) inhibitors such as entacapone (Comtan) and tolcapone (Tasmar); anticholinergics such as trihexyphenidyl (Artane) and benztropine mesylate (Cogentin); and amantadine (Gocovri).

Please consult your healthcare practitioner or a knowledgeable cannabis healthcare provider who can review your medications prior to starting cannabis therapy and continue to monitor you during the duration of treatment. See chart 5 on page 116 for possible CBD interactions.

Post-Traumatic Stress Disorder (PTSD)

While many tend to equate post-traumatic stress disorder (PTSD) with combat veterans, the fact is that PTSD is a mental health disorder that can afflict anyone who has experienced a traumatic event. The symptoms normally start within a month of the event, but it is not unheard of for victims to experience the first symptoms months after the event. It is estimated that PTSD affects approximately 10 percent of people at some point in life.

For many PTSD patients, rest and good self-care is sufficient to work through the symptoms of this disorder. For others, the symptoms may worsen with time and last for years. According to the Mayo Clinic, "PTSD symptoms are generally grouped into four types: Intrusive memories, avoidance, negative changes in thinking and mood, and changes in physical and emotional reactions. Symptoms can vary over time or from person to person."[76]

It has been discovered that the endocannabinoid system (ECS) plays an important role in regulation of emotional behavior and facilitating the synaptic processes that determine learning, especially those related to a potentially traumatic experience.[77] Thus, cannabinoids can likely play a beneficial role in treating PTSD.

A 2018 study published in *Frontiers in Neuroscience*, subtitled "From Bench Research to Confirmation in Human Trials," offers a remarkably thorough look at the potential of CBD in treating this potentially devastating disorder. The study explores the results of animal research with CBD and offers insights into human use of the cannabinoid for treatment of PTSD. While it seems that CBD is most effective for PTSD when administered immediately after the traumatic event, researchers also cited several case studies in which patients responded well to CBD therapy even though the trauma had occurred several years before. In one case, a 10-year-old girl who was sexually abused before the age of 5 was given a dose of CBD (12 to 25 mg once a day) and had improved sleep and less anxiety.[78]

There is insufficient research to conclude that CBD alone is the most effective cannabinoid treatment for PTSD. Full-spectrum cannabis may offer additional therapeutic benefit. Patients should be cautious adding THC to the regimen, since THC can sometimes induce anxiety.

Ideal Delivery Method: Different routes of administration will produce different effects. Individuals can choose which option works best for them based on their goals. See chapter 2 for more details on routes of administration. Depending on the severity of the disease, multiple routes of administration may be most effective.

CBD Dosage: Determining dosages can be complicated. Always start low and go slow. Multiple factors need to be considered when developing a CBD treatment plan. Without double-blind human clinical trials to address CBD dosages for certain conditions, we must rely on preclinical (animal) data. It can be difficult to apply dosages from animal studies to humans, and extreme caution must be used. To date, there are no studies that demonstrate CBD dosages for PTSD as a treatment. The US Department of Veterans Affairs has begun a randomized controlled placebo study with CBD at 600 mg twice a day with a completion date of September 30, 2023.[79]

Precautions: Caution should always be taken when an individual begins a CBD regimen, especially if the individual is taking medications or has a history of chronic illnesses.

Commonly Prescribed Drugs and Potential Drug Interactions: Several types of medications may help improve PTSD symptoms. Antidepressants can help with sleep and concentration. Selective serotonin reuptake inhibitors (SSRIs) like Zoloft and Paxil may be prescribed. Antianxiety medications may also be prescribed, but doctors generally prefer these drugs to be prescribed for short-term use since abuse is possible.

Please consult your healthcare practitioner or a knowledgeable cannabis healthcare provider who can review your medications prior to starting cannabis therapy and continue to monitor you during the duration of treatment. See chart 5 on page 116 for possible CBD interactions.

Stroke

Stroke is a serious health issue in the United States, where it is responsible for more than 140,000 deaths each year. According to the most recent statistics, 795,000 people will have a stroke in any given year, and approximately 600,000 will be first-time occurrences. Stroke is the leading cause of serious, long-term disability in the United States.

There are three types of stroke: ischemic, hemorrhagic, and transient ischemic attack. Ischemic stroke accounts for 87 percent of all strokes and occurs when a clot blocks a blood vessel. Hemorrhagic stroke occurs when a weakened blood vessel ruptures and bleeds. Transient ischemic attack (TIA) is often called a "mini stroke" and occurs when there is a temporary blood clot. Ischemic and TIA strokes may be benefitted by CBD therapy.

The possibility of using CBD in the treatment of stroke emerged in the early part of this century. A 2010 study noted the possible benefit of CBD for stroke victims. "In the past five years, an increasing number of publications have focused on the discovery of the anti-inflammatory, anti-oxidant, and neuroprotective effects of CBD. In particular, CBD exerts positive pharmacological effects in ischemic stroke . . ."[80] The researchers also noted that CBD "has a potent and long-lasting neuroprotective effect when administered both pre- and post-ischemia."[81] This would imply that CBD could be an excellent protecting supplement for those at risk of stroke. One study concluded, "It is to be hoped that cannabidiol will have a palliative action and open new therapeutic possibilities for treating cerebrovascular disorders."[82]

Ideal Delivery Method: Different routes of administration will produce different effects. Individuals can choose which option works best for them based on their goals. See chapter 2 for more details on routes of administration. Depending on the severity of the disease, multiple routes of administration may be most effective.

CBD Dosage: Determining dosages can be complicated. Always start low and go slow. Multiple factors need to be considered when developing a CBD treatment plan. Without double-blind human clinical trials to address CBD dosages for certain conditions, we must rely on preclinical (animal) data. It can be difficult to apply dosages from animal studies to humans, and extreme caution must be used. To date, there are no studies that demonstrate CBD dosages for stroke. Most patients are using CBD for symptom management, particularly spasticity. Titrate up slowly, and use the minimal amount of CBD that can give relief from stroke symptoms.

Precautions: Caution should always be taken when an individual begins a CBD regimen, especially if the individual is taking medications or has a history of chronic illnesses.

Commonly Prescribed Drugs and Potential Drug Interactions: For an ischemic stroke, time is of the essence, and most medications will be administered at the hospital. The results of each stroke will determine what poststroke medications will be prescribed. Physical therapy may also be prescribed. Poststroke medications may include blood thinners such as dabigatran, apixaban, and rivaroxaban or antiplatelet drugs such as aspirin, dipyridamole, and clopidogrel. Antihypertensives to help control high blood pressure and cholesterol-lowering agents called statins may also be used.

Please consult your healthcare practitioner or a knowledgeable cannabis healthcare provider who can review your medications prior to starting cannabis therapy and continue to monitor you during the duration of treatment. See chart 5 on page 116 for possible CBD interactions.

Traumatic Brain Injury (TBI)

A traumatic brain injury (TBI) occurs when an external force injures the brain. This force could come from sudden deceleration, causing the brain to slam into the skull, or it could be due to rapid acceleration, causing the brain to move backward and make damaging contact with the skull. It should come as no surprise that the most common cause of TBI is transportation accidents, particularly on motorbikes. Child and domestic abuse are also frequently listed causes of TBI. Worldwide, TBI accounts for approximately 10 million deaths annually.

As with ischemic stroke, researchers were quick to recognize the potential of the endocannabinoid system in treating TBI. An extensive review published in 2017 concluded, "Overall, the abundant and growing pre-clinical research suggests that the [ECS] system possesses many promising targets for new and existing drugs that may ameliorate diverse TBI pathology."[83]

Most research has looked at the effects of THC on TBI, but anecdotal accounts point to CBD as a helpful post-TBI medication. Santa Monica doctor Allan Frankel believes that incorporating small amounts of CBD as a daily nutritional supplement can be a sensible adjunct to regular therapy. He cites the case of a 45-year-old woman who, after a car accident, was having cognitive issues and difficulties with memory. Within four to six weeks of adding CBD, this patient had cognitively improved and her memory had returned to normal.[84]

TBI patients are encouraged to review the literature to determine if CBD is appropriate. A good summary is available at the website Key to Cannabis.[85]

Ideal Delivery Method: Different routes of administration will produce different effects. Individuals can choose which option works best for them based on their goals. See chapter 2 for more details on routes of administration. Depending on the severity of the disease, multiple routes of administration may be most effective.

CBD Dosage: Determining dosages can be complicated. Multiple factors need to be considered when developing a CBD treatment plan. Without double-blind human clinical trials to address CBD dosages for certain conditions, we must rely on preclinical (animal) data. It can be difficult to apply dosages from animal studies to humans, and extreme caution must be used. To date, there are no studies that demonstrate CBD dosages for TBIs as a treatment. Most patients are using CBD for symptom management. Titrate up slowly, and use the minimal amount of CBD that can give relief from TBI symptoms.

Precautions: Caution should always be taken when an individual begins a CBD regimen, especially if the individual is taking medications or has a history of chronic illnesses.

Commonly Prescribed Drugs and Potential Drug Interactions: TBI is an exceedingly complex injury to treat. The severity of injury can differ widely, as can the symptoms. Basically, there are three categories of conventional medications: anticonvulsants, antidepressants, and anti-psychotics. Pain medications and motor system medications are also commonly prescribed.

Please consult your healthcare practitioner or a knowledgeable cannabis healthcare provider who can review your medications prior to starting cannabis therapy and continue to monitor you during the duration of treatment. See chart 5 on page 116 for possible CBD interactions.

CHAPTER FOUR

CBD FOR PETS

With so much positive feedback on the use of CBD in humans, it was inevitable, especially in Western cultures, that pet lovers would begin to wonder if CBD could be good for their dogs or cats. While research with CBD and pets is sketchy, it is interesting to remember that for years dogs have been used in marijuana research, but primarily drug abuse research. Indirect research with CBD and animals is starting to emerge as a result of preclinical studies with rodents. But direct information is lacking. So, caution is recommended, keeping in mind that our pets may have all the same parts that we do, but their physiologies are different. Proceed slowly, and keep a careful eye on your pets as you begin administering CBD.

Dosage Guidelines

There are several different delivery methods for pet CBD: tincture, capsules, treats, and balm. The method you choose will depend on your goal. Treats and balm can be used on an as-needed basis. For example, if your pet experiences anxiety during thunderstorms, providing a CBD treat or rubbing the balm on the inside of the pet's ear can provide some relief. CBD balm is also excellent for your pet's skin conditions, but be certain to take plenty of time in applying the balm to the skin. Your pet will lick the area, and you want to be sure that most of the balm has been absorbed where it will do the most good. If your pet's problem is longer term and more systemic—arthritis, for example—then you will want CBD in tincture or capsule form.

FACTORS THAT INFLUENCE DOSAGE

The factors that influence pet dosage are similar to human factors: age, weight, medication history, and route of administration.

Age: Older dogs may require slightly higher doses of CBD in order to obtain the same level of relief as younger canines. This is because the dog's physiology is slowing. You may also want to use CBD treats as a means to provide your pet with the optimum daily dose.

Weight: Common sense tells us that a 20-pound dog will need less CBD than a 50-pound dog, so keep this in mind as you explore various brands. Many pet products are formulated with the pet's size in mind, and products are packaged according to various size ranges, with higher concentrations for larger pets. Higher-end CBD pet products have dosing charts available, and, for tinctures, the dropper will be labeled. Nearly all CBD pet product manufacturers provide dosing charts and advice online.

Medication history: You need to consider CBD interaction with other drugs that your pet may be using, in particular drugs that metabolize in the liver. This is because CBD can affect the enzymes that metabolize drugs in the liver. Your vet will be able to tell you if this might be a concern.

Route of administration: Just as with humans, CBD for pets comes in a variety of delivery methods. Included are capsules, tinctures, balm/salve, and edibles. Administering medications to a pet can be a challenge, and if higher doses of CBD are required, it may require some combination of available delivery forms. Most pets will be interested in the edible forms of CBD, but remember that the CBD will pass through the digestive system and the liver, so accurate dosing could be difficult. Similarly, tinctures may be added to food, but this will reduce the dosing accuracy. There are balms or salves with CBD that can be applied to the inside of the ear. For regular dosing, capsules may provide the best means of administration.

STARTING LOW

Just as with humans, the smart way to proceed with CBD and pets is to start low and go slow. CBD is generally safe, but it is an active compound that can have a profound impact. Since dogs and cats can't tell us how they are feeling, it is up to us to monitor their reactions carefully. Do not begin your pet's CBD therapy at the highest level recommended by the product manufacturer. Build up to that level slowly, and be sure you can monitor your pet's response.

WHEN TO START WITH A HIGH DOSE

For the most part, large dosing of pets with CBD is not particularly productive. In fact, it can become counterproductive, making your pet extremely lethargic. (This is one of the mysteries of CBD—at low levels it can energize, and at higher levels it can cause lethargy.) There is some preliminary research pointing to CBD as a possible antibiotic, and using CBD in this way would require large dosing. But you will want to research this carefully before proceeding. Similarly, you may read about high dosing of cannabis to treat cancer in pets (and humans), but most likely this is referring to cannabis oil that has delta-9 THC. You will need to explore whether you can legally obtain this cannabis oil in your state and then do careful research about the oil and its effects on pets.

Dosage Chart

An average range for dosing pets is 1 to 5 mg per every 10 pounds of weight. If giving tinctures, check the manufacturer's suggested dosing. Just like with humans, start low and go slow.

This chart gives you a handy reference point. Start by locating your pet's weight in the left-hand column, then follow across in that row to the correct column to determine the proper dosing for five different doses of CBD. For example, starting with a low dose of 1 mg/lb, if your pet weighs 35 pounds, locate that weight in the left-hand column, then follow the row across to see the correct dose is 35 mg. If your pet weighs 33 pounds, it would be 33 x 1 mg = 33 mg. Rounding off is acceptable, and dosing may end up dependent on available products. You may want to start with half the recommended dose and monitor your pet. It is also recommended that the total dose be split in half and given 12 hours apart. If you are treating pain, consider dosing every 8 hours and increasing to the maximum dose tolerated by your pet as rapidly as you can.

CHART 4: Low and Slow for Pets

WEIGHT OF PET IN LBS	DOSE IS 1 MG PER LB	DOSE IS 2 MG PER LB	DOSE IS 3 MG PER LB	DOSE IS 4 MG PER LB	DOSE IS 5 MG PER LB
5	5 mg	10 mg	15 mg	20 mg	25 mg
10	10 mg	20 mg	30 mg	40 mg	50 mg

WEIGHT OF PET IN LBS	DOSE IS 1 MG PER LB	DOSE IS 2 MG PER LB	DOSE IS 3 MG PER LB	DOSE IS 4 MG PER LB	DOSE IS 5 MG PER LB
15	15 mg	30 mg	45 mg	60 mg	75 mg
20	20 mg	40 mg	60 mg	80 mg	100 mg
25	25 mg	50 mg	75 mg	100 mg	125 mg
30	30 mg	60 mg	90 mg	120 mg	150 mg
35	35 mg	70 mg	105 mg	140 mg	175 mg
40	40 mg	80 mg	120 mg	160 mg	200 mg
45	45 mg	90 mg	135 mg	180 mg	225 mg
50	50 mg	100 mg	150 mg	200 mg	250 mg
55	55 mg	110 mg	165 mg	220 mg	275 mg
60	60 mg	120 mg	180 mg	240 mg	300 mg
65	65 mg	130 mg	195 mg	260 mg	325 mg
70	70 mg	140 mg	210 mg	280 mg	350 mg
75	75 mg	150 mg	225 mg	300 mg	375 mg
80	80 mg	160 mg	240 mg	320 mg	400 mg
85	85 mg	170 mg	255 mg	340 mg	425 mg
90	90 mg	180 mg	270 mg	360 mg	450 mg
95	95 mg	190 mg	285 mg	380 mg	475 mg
100	100 mg	200 mg	300 mg	400 mg	500 mg

Pet Ailments That May Respond to CBD

If your dog or cat has any of the following ailments, you may want to consider CBD therapy:

- Anxiety

- Arthritis—this is the primary use of CBD in pets

- Autoimmune disorders

- Cancer

- Congenital orthopedic conditions (hip dysplasia, spinal scoliosis)

- Digestive and gastrointestinal ailments

- Epilepsy

- Inflammation

- Pain from injuries, surgery, or disease

- Skin disorders

- Stress

CBD Interaction with Commonly Prescribed Drugs

If you are using oral CBD—capsules, tinctures, or edibles—this chart will provide information on how the CBD interacts with other medications and how it is metabolized in the body.

Oral CBD is metabolized in the liver and often uses the same pathway as other drugs as it is metabolized. This situation can increase (↑) or decrease (↓) the effects of CBD or the competing drug and requires monitoring on the part of the patient and healthcare providers.

This chart is for reference purposes only and applies only to oral CBD, not inhaled or topical. Research is incomplete with respect to CBD's interactions with conventional medications. Please consult your healthcare practitioner or a knowledgeable cannabis healthcare provider who can review your medications prior to starting cannabis therapy and continue to monitor you during the duration of treatment.

The following information was extracted from Lexicomp (2019) and Wolters Kluwer Clinical Drug Information (version 4.6.0).

CHART 5: CBD Interaction with Commonly Prescribed Drugs

DRUG	BRANDS	METABOLISM PATHWAY VIA LIVER
ABACAVIR/ DOLUTEGRAVIR/ LAMIVUDINE	Triumeq	Same
ACAMPROSATE	Campral	Unknown
ADALIMUMAB	Humira	Unknown
ALEMTUZUMAB	Campath, Lemtrada	Unknown
ALOSETRON	Lotronex	Same
ALPRAZOLAM	Xanax	Same
AMANTADINE	Gocovri	Different pathway
AMITRIPTYLINE	Elavil	Same
AMOXICILLIN	Moxatag	Unknown
APIXABAN	Eliquis	Same
APREPITANT	Emend	Same
ASPIRIN	Multiple brands	Same
ATORVASTATIN	Lipitor	Same
AZATHIOPRINE	Azasan	Unknown

INTERACTION WITH CBD	NOTES
None known	Monitor.
None known	Monitor.
None known	Monitor.
None known	Monitor.
None known	Monitor.
CBD may ↑ effects	Monitor for ↑ side effects of drug. Use extreme caution with CBD.
None known	Monitor.
None known	CBD has potential to ↑ effects of amitriptyline.
None known	Monitor.
None known	Monitor for increased bleeding.
Has the potential to ↑ the effects of CBD	Monitor for ↑ in effects of CBD.
None known	Monitor.
None known	Monitor.
None known	Monitor.

DRUG	BRANDS	METABOLISM PATHWAY VIA LIVER
BACLOFEN	Lioresal, Gablofen	Unknown
BENZTROPINE MESYLATE	Cogentin	Same
BICTEGRAVIR/ EMTRICITABINE/ TENOFOVIR ALAFENAMIDE	Biktarvy	Same
BUPRENORPHINE	Belbuca, Probuphine, Buprenex, Butrans	Same
BUSPIRONE	BuSpar	Same
CAPSAICIN	Capsaicin	Different
CARBAMAZEPINE	Tegretol, Equetro, and others	Same
CARBIDOPA-LEVODOPA	Duopa, Sinemet, Rytary	Unknown
CEFUROXIME	Zinacef, Ceftin	Unknown
CELECOXIB	Celebrex	Same
CITALOPRAM	Celexa	Same
CLONAZEPAM	Klonopin	Same

INTERACTION WITH CBD	NOTES
May ↑ drug effect	Monitor for ↑ side effects of drug. Use extreme caution with CBD.
None known	Monitor.
None known	Monitor.
May ↑ drug effect	Monitor and consider dosage adjustments with concurrent use.
May ↑ effect of buspirone	Monitor and consider dosage adjustments with concurrent use.
None known	Monitor.
May ↑ drug effect	Monitor and consider dosage adjustments with concurrent use.
None known	Monitor.
None known	Monitor.
None known	Monitor.
None known	Monitor for potential ↑ drug effect with CBD use.
CBD may ↑ effects	Monitor for ↑ side effects of drug. Use extreme caution with CBD.

DRUG	BRANDS	METABOLISM PATHWAY VIA LIVER
CLOPIDOGREL	Plavix	Same
CYCLOBENZAPRINE	Amrix, Fexmid	Same
CYCLOPHOSPHAMIDE	Cytoxan	Same
CYCLOSPORINE	Restasis, Sandimmune	Same
DABIGATRAN ETEXILATE	Pradaxa	Same
DEXAMETHASONE	Ozurdex, DexPak 6	Same
DEXTROMETHORPHAN	Multiple including Tussin Cough (DM only), Scot-Tussin Diabetes CF, Robitussin ER, Tussin Maximum Strength	Same
DIAZEPAM	Valium	Same
DIMETHYL FUMARATE	Tecfidera	Unknown
DIPHENOXYLATE/ ATROPINE	Lomotil	Same
DISULFIRAM	Antabuse	Same
DOLUTEGRAVIR/ RILPIVIRINE	Juluca	Same

INTERACTION WITH CBD	NOTES
None known	Monitor for increased bleeding.
Potential for CBD to ↑ effects of cyclobenzaprine	Monitor and consider dosage adjustments with concurrent use.
None known	Available in tablets and IV. Monitor.
Potential for CBD to ↑ cyclosporine	Monitor.
None known	Monitor for increased bleeding.
CBD has potential to ↑ effects of dexamethasone	Monitor.
Unknown	Monitor for potential ↑ drug effect with CBD use.
CBD may ↑ effects	Monitor for ↑ side effects of drug. Use extreme caution with CBD.
None known	Monitor.
None known	Potential for CBD to ↑ diphenoxylate and atropine. Monitor for increased drug effect.
None known	Interaction is clinically insignificant.
None known	Monitor.

DRUG	BRANDS	METABOLISM PATHWAY VIA LIVER
DONEPEZIL	Aricept	Same
DOXYCYCLINE	Doxy-100, Oracea, Targadox	Unknown
DRONABINOL	Marinol	Same
DULOXETINE	Cymbalta	Same
EDARAVONE	Radicava	Unknown
EFAVIRENZ/ EMTRICITABINE/ TENOFOVIR DISOPROXIL FUMARATE	Atripla	Same
ELUXADOLINE	Viberzi, Truberzi	Different pathways
ELVITEGRAVIR/ COBICISTAT/ EMTRICITABINE/ TENOFOVIR ALAFENAMIDE	Genvoya	Same
ELVITEGRAVIR/ COBICISTAT/ EMTRICITABINE/ TENOFOVIR DISOPROXIL FUMARATE	Stribild	Same

INTERACTION WITH CBD	NOTES
None known	Monitor.
None known	Monitor.
CBD has the potential to ↓ the side effects from dronabinol but not the effectiveness	Monitor.
CBD may ↓ drug effect	Monitor effect.
None known	Monitor for potential ↑ drug effect.
CBD may ↑ effects	Monitor for ↑ side effects of drug. Use caution with CBD.
None known	Monitor.
Potential to ↑ the effects of CBD	Monitor for ↑ the effects of CBD. Consider dose reduction of CBD.
Potential to ↑ the effects of CBD	Monitor for ↑ the effects of CBD. Consider dose reduction of CBD.

DRUG	BRANDS	METABOLISM PATHWAY VIA LIVER
EMTRICITABINE/ RILPIVIRINE/ TENOFOVIR ALAFENAMIDE	Odefsey	Same
EMTRICITABINE/ RILPIVIRINE/ TENOFOVIR DISOPROXIL FUMARATE	Complera	Same
ENTACAPONE	Comtan	Same
ESCITALOPRAM	Lexapro	Same
ESZOPICLONE	Lunesta	Same
ETANERCEPT	Enbrel	Unknown
FENTANYL	Duragesic	Same
FINGOLIMOD	Gilenya	Same
FLUOXETINE	Prozac	Same
GABAPENTIN	Neurontin	Unknown
GALANTAMINE	Razadyne	Same

INTERACTION WITH CBD	NOTES
None known	Monitor.
None known	Monitor.
CBD may ↑ effects	Monitor for potential ↑ drug effect with CBD use.
None known	Monitor for potential ↑ drug effect with CBD use.
None known	CBD has potential to ↑ effects of eszopiclone. Monitor.
None known	Monitor.
CBD may ↑ effects	Monitor for ↑ side effects of drug. Use caution with CBD.
None known	Monitor.
None known	Monitor for potential ↑ drug effect with CBD use.
Levels of gabapentin may ↑ with CBD	Monitor.
None known	Monitor.

DRUG	BRANDS	METABOLISM PATHWAY VIA LIVER
GLATIRAMER ACETATE	Copaxone	Unknown
GRANISETRON	Sustol	Same
HALOPERIDOL	Haldol	Same
HYDROCODONE	Vicodin	Same
HYDROXYCHLOROQUINE	Plaquenil	Unknown
HYDROXYZINE	Hydroxyzine	Unknown
IBUPROFEN	Advil, Motrin, many others	Same
INFLIXIMAB	Remicade	Unknown
ISOCARBOXAZID	Marplan	Different pathways
LEVETIRACETAM	Roweepra, Keppra	Same
LINACLOTIDE	Linzess	Unknown
LORAZEPAM	Ativan	Unknown

INTERACTION WITH CBD	NOTES
None known	Monitor.
CBD has the potential to ↑ the effects of granisetron	Monitor and use caution.
Potential for CBD to ↑ haloperidol	Monitor.
CBD has potential to ↑ the effects of hydrocodone	Monitor and use caution. Patient may be able to ↓ hydroco-done with CBD use.
None known	Monitor.
May ↑ effect of hydroxyzine	Monitor.
None known	Monitor.
None known	Monitor.
Isocarboxazid may ↑ effects of CBD	Monitor and consider CBD dose adjustments.
Unknown	Potential for CBD to ↑ levetiracetam. Monitor for increased drug effect.
None known	Monitor.
CBD may ↑ effects of lorazepam	Use extreme caution with CBD.

DRUG	BRANDS	METABOLISM PATHWAY VIA LIVER
LOSARTAN	Cozaar	Same
LUBIPROSTONE	Amitiza	Unknown
MELOXICAM	Mobic, Viviodex	Same
MERCAPTOPURINE	Purixan	Unknown
METHADONE	Diskets, Methadone Intensol, Methadose, and Dolophine	Same
METHOTREXATE	Otrexup, Xatmep, Trexall	Same
MILNACIPRAN	Savella	Unknown
MITOXANTRONE	Mitoxantrone	Different
MYCOPHENOLATE	CellCept, Myfortic	Different pathways
NABILONE	Cesamet	Unknown
NALTREXONE	Vivitrol, Revia	Unknown
NAPROXEN	Aleve, Naprosyn, many others	Same
NATALIZUMAB	Tysabri	Unknown

INTERACTION WITH CBD	NOTES
None known	Monitor.
None known	Monitor.
None known	Monitor.
None known	Monitor.
CBD may ↑ drug effect of methadone	Monitor and consider dosage adjustments with concurrent use.
None known	Monitor.
None known	Monitor.
None known	Monitor.
None known	Monitor.
CBD has the potential to ↓ the side effects from nabilone but not the effectiveness	Monitor.
None known	Monitor.
None known	Monitor.
None known	Monitor.

DRUG	BRANDS	METABOLISM PATHWAY VIA LIVER
NORTRIPTYLINE	Pamelor	Same
OCRELIZUMAB	Ocrevus	Unknown
OLANZAPINE	Zyprexa	Same
ONDANSETRON	Zofran	Same
OXCARBAZEPINE	Octellar XR, Trileptal	Same
OXYCODONE	Roxicodone, Xtampza, Oxaydo	Same
PALONOSETRON	Aloxi	Same
PAROXETINE	Paxil	Same
PHENELZINE	Nardil	Different pathways
PRAMIPEXOLE	Mirapex	Unknown
PREDNISONE	Deltasone, Rayos	Same
PREGABALIN	Lyrica	Unknown

INTERACTION WITH CBD	NOTES
None known	CBD has potential to ↑ effects of nortriptyline.
None known	Monitor.
Potential for CBD to ↑ olanzapine	Monitor and consider dosage adjustments with concurrent use. Use with caution.
CBD has the potential to ↑ the effects of ondansetron	Monitor and use caution.
None known	Monitor.
CBD has potential to ↑ the effects of oxycodone	Monitor and use caution. Patient may be able to ↓ oxycodone with CBD use.
CBD has the potential to ↑ the effects of palonosetron	Monitor and use caution.
None known	Monitor for potential ↑ drug effect with CBD use.
Phenelzine may ↑ effects of CBD	Monitor and consider CBD dose adjustments.
None known	Monitor.
None known	Monitor.
None known	Monitor for potential ↑ drug effect with CBD use.

DRUG	BRANDS	METABOLISM PATHWAY VIA LIVER
PROPRANOLOL	Inderal LA or XL, Hemangeol	Same
QUETIAPINE	Seroquel XR, Seroquel	Same
QUINIDINE	Nudexta	Same
RIFAXIMIN	Xifaxan	Same
RILUZOLE	Rilutek	Same
RISPERIDONE	Risperdal	Same
RIVASTIGMINE	Exelon	Unknown
RIZATRIPTAN	Maxalt	Unknown
ROPINIROLE	Requip	Same
ROSUVASTATIN	Crestor	Same
SELEGILINE	Eldepryl, Zelapar	Same
SERTRALINE	Zoloft	Same

INTERACTION WITH CBD	NOTES
None known	Monitor for ↓ of drug effect.
May ↑ effect of quetiapine	Monitor for ↑ drug effect. Use with caution.
Unknown	Monitor for potential ↑ drug effect with CBD use.
None known	Monitor.
None known	Monitor for potential ↓ drug effect with CBD use.
Potential for CBD to ↑ risperidone	Monitor and consider dose adjustments. Use with caution.
None known	Monitor.
None known	Monitor.
CBD may ↓ drug effect	Monitor for decreased drug effect.
None known	Monitor.
None known	Monitor.
None known	Monitor for potential ↑ drug effect with CBD use.

DRUG	BRANDS	METABOLISM PATHWAY VIA LIVER
SIPONIMOD	Mayzent	Same
SUMATRIPTAN	Imitrex, several other brands	Unknown
TEMAZEPAM	Restoril	Same
TERIFLUNOMIDE	Aubagio	Same
TETRABENAZINE	Xenazine	Same
TOLCAPONE	Tasmar	Same
TOPIRAMATE	Trokendi XR, Qudexy XR, Topamax	Unknown
TRAMADOL	Ultram	Same
TRANYLCYPROMINE	Parnate	Same
TRAZODONE	Desyrel	Same
TRIHEXYPHENIDYL	Artane	Unknown
VENLAFAXINE	Effexor	Unknown

INTERACTION WITH CBD	NOTES
None known	Monitor.
None known	Monitor.
None known	CBD has potential to ↑ effects of temazepam. Monitor.
None known	Monitor.
CBD may ↑ tetrabenazine	Monitor.
Levels of tolcapone may ↑ with CBD	Monitor for ↑ side effects.
Levels of topiramate may ↑ with CBD	Monitor for ↑ side effects.
None known	CBD may ↑ effects of tramadol. Monitor.
Tranylcypromine may ↑ effects of CBD	Monitor and consider CBD dose adjustments.
Unknown	CBD has potential to ↑ the effects of trazadone.
None known	Monitor.
None known	CBD has potential to ↑ venlafaxine.

Recommended CBD Brands

CHART 6: Recommended CBD Brands

BRAND & WEBSITE	OFFERINGS	COST RANGE
BASIC JANE www.basicjane.com	Tp, FS	**$12.00 to $54.00** Price-saving bundles available
BLUEBIRD BOTANICALS www.bluebirdbotanicals.com	C, T	**$24.99 to $119.95**
CIRCLE LABS www.circlelabs.co	T, Tr, FS	**$38.00 to $650.00**
CW BOTANICALS www.charlottesweb.com	C, T, Tp, E, I, FS, P	**$39.99 to $164.99**
GREEN ROADS www.greenroadsworld.com	C, T, Tp, E, I, P	**$26.99 to $162.99** (Isolates only)

Cost Range based on tincture products including the company's lowest potency tincture (normally around 7 mg to 15 mg) to its highest potency (around 33 mg to 60 mg), in 30 ml-bottle tinctures. Full-spectrum unless otherwise noted.

WHERE TO BUY	WHY RECOMMENDED
Online	*A young company focusing on topicals, Basic Jane carries high quality and reasonably priced products.*
Online	*One of the first hemp extract companies, Bluebird sells no-frills, quality CBD products.*
Online	*Circle Labs uses high standards in plant genetics, regenerative and organic farming conditions, and cold-press processing to preserve the flower.*
Online, CBD stores	*Charlotte's Web is legendary in the CBD world. They consistently prepare quality product at competitive prices.*
Online or at spas and health food stores around the country	*Founded by a pharmacist, Green Roads offers an excellent array of products.*

BRAND & WEBSITE	OFFERINGS	COST RANGE
LAZARUS NATURALS www.lazarusnaturals.com	C, T, Tp, P, FS, I	$24.00 to $64.00
MISSION FARMS www.missionfarmscbd.com	T, TP, I, FS,	$29.00 to $99.00
MYRIAM'S HOPE HEMP www.myriamshopehemp.com	T, Tp, FS, P	$47.50 to $160.00
PURE HEMP www.purehempbotanicals. com	C, T, FS, I, E, P	$24.95 to $124.95
RE BOTANICALS www.rebotanicals.com	C, T, FS, P	$49.99 to $139.99
TRUE FARMA www.truefarmacbd.com	C, T, Tp, Tr, E, I, FS, P	N/A

WHERE TO BUY	WHY RECOMMENDED
Online and numerous stores nationwide. Store locator on website.	They offer high-quality products (isolates and full-spectrum) and discounts for veterans, low-income, and long-term disability patients.
Online	This Oregon-based manufacturer packages its CBD with an emphasis on goal—e.g., Rest CBD Cream, Relieve CBD Oil. The company provides trial-size bottles with a money-back guarantee.
Online	This online company offers CBDa and CBD tinctures. They have a Compassion Program for seniors, veterans, and low-income patients.
Online	Known for their excellent transparency and wide range of products, this company receives consistently strong reviews online.
Online and at shops nationwide. Website has a store locator.	Their topicals have essential oils and are packaged in a roller-ball container for easy application.
Online	If you want to shop for a variety of CBD products on one website, True Farma is your place. They sell numerous products from different manufacturers, including CBD vape pens, CBD patches, and bundles.

RESOURCES

Websites

PROJECT CBD
Possibly the best online source for information on CBD. Website includes information for those new to CBD as well as detailed reports on CBD research. www.projectcbd.org

REALM OF CARING
The RoC grew out of the parents' movement to acquire CBD for their children. It has grown into a multi-faceted organization with education modules, research, and a patient care team. www.theroc.us

CNN WEED SPECIALS WITH DR. SANJAY GUPTA
See the documentaries that lit a fire under the CBD movement. https://www.cnn.com/2013/08/08/health/gupta-changed-mind-marijuana/index.html

CBD OIL USERS
A helpful website with education, product reviews, and buying advice. https://cbdoilusers.com

HEALER
Dr. Dustin Sulak is a preeminent physician in the medical cannabis realm. His website is packed with helpful information, including information on dosing. https://healer.com

MARY'S PUBLICATIONS
Timely news on research and basic information on medical cannabis. This website is sponsored by Mary's Brands of Denver, Colorado, and the materials are written and prepared by Alice O'Leary Randall, the author of this book. www.maryspubs.com

Books

Cannabis Pharmacy by Michael Backes (2017)
A very useful book, although it is cannabis centered. It has a large collection of disease categories and recommendations for treatment with cannabis.

Cannabis Revealed by Bonni Goldstein (2016)
Dr. Goldstein specializes in cannabis medicine in Los Angeles. This book is easy to read and highly educational.

CBD: A Patient's Guide to Medicinal Cannabis
by Leonard Leinow and Juliana Birnbaum (2017)
Highly informative book with plenty of tips for using CBD.

Healing with CBD by Eileen Konieczny (2018)
Eileen Konieczny is a registered nurse and former president of the American Cannabis Nurses Association.

Pet Resources

CANNABIS DOG DOSING CHART
Helpful guidance for using CBD with your pets. https://s3-us-west
-2.amazonaws.com/cannabisfreebies/DOG+Cannabis+HempRx+
Dosing+Chart.pdf

CANNABIS OIL FOR DOGS: EVERYTHING YOU NEED TO KNOW
Informative website on the use of CBD in pets. https://www.petmd.com
/dog/general-health/cannabis-oil-dogs-everything-you-need-know

CBD DOSAGE CALCULATOR
Useful information with a calculator. https://www.innovetpet.com/pages
/cbd-dosing-calculator

8 THINGS YOU NEED TO KNOW ABOUT DOGS AND MARIJUANA
A helpful webpage at CanineJournal.Com. https://www.caninejournal
.com/dogs-and-marijuana

NOTES

[1] Lopez, German. "New Data Shows Drug Overdose Deaths Fell In 2018. But There's a Big Catch." *Vox*. July 17, 2019. https://www.vox.com/science-and-health /2019/7/17/20698040/opioid-epidemic-drug-overdose-deaths-2018.

[2] Gallup. "Americans Prefer Drug-Free Pain Management over Opioids." Accessed September 14, 2019. https://news.gallup.com/reports/217676/americans-prefer -drug-free-pain-management-opioids.aspx.

[3] Marinac, Jacqueline S. et al. "Herbal Products and Dietary Supplements: A Survey of Use, Attitudes, and Knowledge Among Older Adults." *Journal of the American Osteopathic Association* 107 (January 2007): 13–23. https://jaoa.org /article.aspx?articleid=2093317.

[4] Backes, Michael. *Cannabis Pharmacy*. New York: Black Dog & Leventhal, 2014.

[5] Merriam-Webster. "Psychoactive." Accessed September 14, 2019. https://www .merriam-webster.com/dictionary/psychoactive.

[6] Hudak, John. "The Farm Bill, Hemp Legalization and the Status of CBD: An Explainer." Brookings. Last modified December 14, 2019. https://www.brookings .edu/blog/fixgov/2018/12/14/the-farm-bill-hemp-and-cbd-explainer/.

[7] Backes, *Cannabis Pharmacy*, 184.

[8] Backes, *Cannabis Pharmacy*, 184.

[9] Backes, *Cannabis Pharmacy*, 206–25.

[10] Resing, Charlotte. "Marijuana Legalization Is a Racial Justice Issue." ACLU. Last modified April 20, 2019. https://www.aclu.org/blog/criminal-law-reform/drug -law-reform/marijuana-legalization-racial-justice-issue.

[11] Project CBD. "The Endocannabinoid System." Accessed August 10, 2019. https:// www.projectcbd.org/science/endocannabinoid-system-0.

[12] It is important to remember these are not necessarily all studies with CBD but rather scientific articles that mention CBD. Patients are encouraged to do disease-specific searches using Google Scholar.

[13] Crippa, Jose Alexandre S. et al. "Is Cannabidiol the Ideal Drug to Treat Non-Motor Parkinson's Disease Symptoms?" *European Archives of Psychiatry and Clinical Neuroscience* 269 (Februrary 2019): 121–133. doi:10.1007/s00406-019-00982-6.

[14] Shannon, S., N. Lewis, H. Lee, and S. Hughes. "Cannabidiol in Anxiety and Sleep: A Large Case Series." *The Permanente Journal* 23 (2019): 18–041. doi:10.7812/TPP /18-041.

[15] Boehnke, Kevin F. et al. "Cannabis Use Preferences and Decision-Making Among a Cross-Sectional Cohort of Medical Cannabis Patients with Chronic Pain." *The Journal of Pain* (May 2019). doi:10.1016/j.jpain.2019.05.009.

[16] Somerset, Sara Brittany. "Can CBD Cause Liver Damage?" *Forbes*. Last modified July 11, 2019. https://www.forbes.com/sites/sarabrittanysomerset/2019/07/11/of -mice-and-men-is-cbd-toxic-to-the-liver/#2b7659743daa.

[17] Health Behavior News Service, part of the Center for Advancing Health. "Chronic Pain Sufferers Likely to Have Anxiety." ScienceDaily. Accessed September 14, 2019. http://www.sciencedaily.com/releases/2013/05/130508213112.htm.

[18] Fitzgibbon, Marie, David P. Finn, and Michelle Roche. "High Times for Painful Blues: The Endocannabinoid System in Pain-Depression Comorbidity." *International Journal of Neuropsychopharmacology* 19, no. 3 (March 2016): pyv095. doi:10.1093/ijnp/pyv095.

[19] Harvard Health Publishing. "The Pain-Anxiety-Depression Connection." Last modified May 20, 2015. https://www.health.harvard.edu/healthbeat/the-pain -anxiety-depression-connection.

[20] De Gregorio, Danilo et al. "Cannabidiol Modulates Serotonergic Transmission and Reverses Both Allodynia and Anxiety-like Behavior in a Model of Neuropathic Pain." *Pain* 160, no. 1 (2019): 136–50. doi:10.1097/j.pain.0000000000001386.

[21] Bonn-Miller, Marcel O. et al. "Labeling Accuracy of Cannabidiol Extracts Sold Online." *JAMA* 318, no. 17 (2017): 1708–09. doi:10.1001/jama.2017.11909.

[22] Hess, C., M. Kramer, and B. Madea. "Topical Application of THC Containing Products Is Not Able to Cause Positive Cannabinoid Finding in Blood or Urine." *Forensic Science International* 272 (March 2017): 68–71. doi:10.1016/j.forsciint.2017.01.008.

[23] Amazon Seller Central. "Drugs & Drug Paraphernalia." Last modified August 8, 2019. https://sellercentral.amazon.com/gp/help/external/help.html?itemID=200164490&language=en-US&ref=efph_200164490_cont_200164330.

[24] National Institutes of Health. "Pharmacogenomics." Last modified October 1, 2017. https://www.nigms.nih.gov/education/Documents/pharmacogenomics1.pdf.

[25] Grim, Ryan. "CNN 'Weed' Documentary Follows Sanjay Gupta's Reversal On Marijuana." *HuffPost*. Last modified August 12, 2013. https://www.huffpost.com/entry/cnn-weed-documentary_n_3741256.

[26] Gonzalez-Cuevas, Gustavo et al. "Unique Treatment Potential of Cannabidiol for the Prevention of Relapse to Drug Use: Preclinical Proof of Principle." *Neuropsychopharmacology* 43 (September 2018): 2036–45. doi:10.1038/s41386-018-0050-8.

[27] De Ternay, Julia et al. "Therapeutic Prospects of Cannabidiol for Alcohol Use Disorder and Alcohol-Related Damages on the Liver and the Brain." *Frontiers in Pharmacology* 10, no. 627 (2019). doi:10.3389/fphar.2019.00627.

[28] Sullum, Jacob. "Does Medical Marijuana Reduce Opioid-Related Deaths or Not?" *Reason*. June 11, 2019. https://reason.com/2019/06/11/does-medical-marijuana-reduce-opioid-related-deaths-or-not/.

[29] Gonzalez-Cuevas, Gustavo et al. "Unique Treatment Potential of Cannabidiol for the Prevention of Relapse to Drug Use: Preclinical Proof of Principle." *Neuropsychopharmacology* 43 (September 2018): 2036–45. doi:10.1038/s41386-018-0050-8.

[30] Dementia Care Central. "Using CBD (Cannabidiol) to Treat the Symptoms of Alzheimer's & Other Dementias." Last modified February 26, 2019. https://www .dementiacarecentral.com/aboutdementia/treating/cbd/.

[31] Schubert, David et al. "Efficacy of Cannabinoids in a Pre-Clinical Drug-Screening Platform for Alzheimer's Disease." *Molecular Neurobiology* (May 2019). doi:10.1007/s12035-019-1637-8.

[32] Giacoppo, Sabrina, and Emanuela Mazzon. "Can Cannabinoids Be a Potential Therapeutic Tool in Amyotrophic Lateral Sclerosis?" *Neural Regeneration Research* 11, no. 12 (December 2016): 1896–99. doi:10.4103/1673-5374.197125.

[33] Anderson, Zac. "Victory for Cathy Jordan, 'Patron Saint' of Florida Medical Marijuana." *Herald-Tribune*. March 24, 2019. https://www.heraldtribune.com /news/20190324/victory-for-cathy-jordan-patron-saint-of-florida-medical -marijuana.

[34] Nahler, Gerhard. "Co-Medication with Cannabidiol May Slow Down the Progression of Motor Neuron Disease: A Case Report." *Journal of General Practice* 5, no. 4. doi:10.4172/2329-9126.1000316.

[35] National Institute of Mental Health. "Any Anxiety Disorder." Last modified November 2017. https://www.nimh.nih.gov/health/statistics/any-anxiety-disorder.shtml.

[36] Shannon, S. et al. "Cannabidiol in Anxiety and Sleep: A Large Case Series." *The Permanente Journal* 23 (2019): 18–41. doi:10.7812/TPP/18-041.

[37] Shannon, "Cannabidiol in Anxiety and Sleep."

[38] Arthritis Foundation. "CBD Guidance for Adults with Arthritis." Accessed September 30, 2019. https://www.arthritis.org/living-with-arthritis/pain -management/chronic-pain/arthritis-foundation-cbd-guidance-for-adults.php.

[39] Ueberall, Michael A., Ute Essner, and Gerhard H. H. Mueller-Schwefe. "Effectiveness and Tolerability of THC:CBD Oromucosal Spray as Add-on Measure in Patients with Severe Chronic Pain: Analysis of 12-Week Open-Label Real-World Data Provided by the German Pain E-Registry." *Journal of Pain Research* 12 (2019): 1577–1604. doi:10.2147/JPR.S192174.

[40] Hammell, D. C. et al. "Transdermal Cannabidiol Reduces Inflammation and Pain-Related Behaviours in a Rat Model of Arthritis." *European Journal of Pain* 20 (October 2015): 936–48. doi:10.1002/ejp.818.

[41] Rath, "CBD Oil."

[42] Pergam, Steven A. et al. "Cannabis Use among Patients at a Comprehensive Cancer Center in a State with Legalized Medicinal and Recreational Use." *Cancer* 123, no. 22 (September 2017): 4488–97. doi:10.1002/cncr.30879.

[43] Darmani, Nissar A. "Delta-9-Tetrahydrocannabinol Differentially Suppresses Cisplatin-Induced Emesis and Indices of Motor Function via Cannabinoid CB1 Receptors in the Least Shrew." *Pharmacology Biochemistry and Behavior* 69, no. 1–2 (May–June 2001): 239–49. doi:10.1016/S0091-3057(01)00531-7;

Darmani, Nissar. 2001. "Δ9-Tetrahydrocannabinol and Synthetic Cannabinoids Prevent Emesis Produced by the Cannabinoid CB1 Receptor Antagonist/Inverse Agonist SR 141716A." *Neuropsychopharmacology* 24, no. 2 (February 2001): 198–203. Doi:10.1016/S0893-133X(00)00197-4;

Kwiatkowska, Magdalena et al. "A Comparative Analysis of the Potential of Cannabinoids and Ondansetron to Suppress Cisplatin-Induced Emesis in the *Suncus Murinus* (House Musk Shrew)." *Psychopharmacology* 174, no. 2 (July 2004): 254–59. doi:10.1007/s00213-003-1739-9;

Sharkey, K. A. et al. "Arvanil, Anandamide And N-arachidonoyl-dopamine (NADA) Inhibit Emesis through Cannabinoid CB1 and Vanilloid TRPV1 Receptors in the Ferret." *European Journal of Neuroscience* 25: 2773–82. doi:10.1111/j.1460-9568.2007.05521.x;

Ray, Andrew P., Seetha Chebolu, and Nissar A. Darmani. "Receptor-Selective Agonists Induce Emesis and Fos Expression in the Brain and Enteric Nervous System of the Least Shrew (*Cryptotis parva*)." *Pharmacology Biochemistry and Behavior* 94, no. 1 (November 2009): 211–18. doi:10.1016/j.pbb.2009.08.010;

Rock, E. M. et al. "Tetrahydrocannabinolic Acid Reduces Nausea-Induced Conditioned Gaping in Rats and Vomiting in *Suncus murinus*." *British Journal of Pharmacology* 170: 641–48. doi:10.1111/bph.12316.

[44] Orwell, George. *1984*, part 3, chapter 1. Accessed September 17, 2019. http://www.george-orwell.org/1984/17.html.

[45] Boehnke, K. F., E. Litinas, and D. J. Clauw. "Medical Cannabis Use Is Associated with Decreased Opiate Medication Use in a Retrospective Cross-Sectional Survey of Patients with Chronic Pain." *The Journal of Pain* 17, no. 6 (June 2016): 739–44. doi:10.1016/j.jpain.2016.03.002.

[46] Tyree, Griffin A. et al. "A Cost-Effectiveness Model for Adjunctive Smoked Cannabis in the Treatment of Chronic Neuropathic Pain." *Cannabis and Cannabinoid Research* 4, no. 1 (2019): 62–72. doi:10.1089/can.2018.0027.

[47] Jagerovic, Nadine, and Laura Hernandez-Folgado. "Cannabinoids and Neuropathic Pain." *Mini Reviews in Medical Chemistry* 3, no. 7 (2003): 765–72. doi:10.2174/1389557033487818.

[48] Diabetes.co.uk. "CBD Compound in Cannabis Could Treat Diabetes, Researchers Suggest." Last modified April 24, 2015. https://www.diabetes.co.uk/news/2015/Apr/cbd-compound-in-cannabis-could-treat-diabetes,-researchers-suggest-95335970.html.

[49] Ward, Sara Jane. "Cannabidiol Inhibits Paclitaxel-Induced Neuropathic Pain Through 5-HT1A Receptors without Diminishing Nervous System Function or Chemotherapy Efficacy." *British Journal of Pharmacology* 171, no. 3 (2014): 636–45. doi:10.1111/bph.12439.

[50] Serpell, M. et al. "A Double-Blind, Randomized, Placebo-Controlled, Parallel Group Study Of THC/CBD Spray in Peripheral Neuropathic Pain Treatment." *European Journal of Pain* 18, no. 7 (August 2014): 999–1012. doi:10.1002/j.1532-2149.2013.00445.x.

[51] Preidt, Robert. "What Drugs Work Best for Diabetic Nerve Pain?" WebMD. Last modified March 24, 2017. https://www.webmd.com/diabetes/news/20170324/what-drugs-work-best-for-diabetic-nerve-pain#1.

[52] Van de Donk, Tine et al. "An Experimental Randomized Study on the Analgesic Effects of Pharmaceutical-Grade Cannabis in Chronic Pain Patients with Fibromyalgia." *Pain* 160, no. 4 (April 2019): 860–69. doi:10.1097/j.pain.0000000000001464.

[53] White, C. M. "A Review of Human Studies Assessing Cannabidiol's (CBD) Therapeutic Actions and Potential." *Journal of Clinical Pharmacology* 59, no. 7 (July 2019): 923–24. doi:10.1002/jcph.1387.

[54] American for Safe Access. "HIV/AIDS & Medical Marijuana." Accessed August 11, 2019. https://www.safeaccessnow.org/hiv-aids#research.

[55] Maor, Y. et al. "Cannabidiol Inhibits Growth and Induces Programmed Cell Death in Kaposi Sarcoma-Associated Herpesvirus-Infected Endothelium." *Genes & Cancer* 3, no. 7–8 (July 2012): 512–20. doi:10.1177/1947601912466556.

[56] Healthline. "HIV Treatments: List of Prescription Medications." Last modified January 2, 2018. https://www.healthline.com/health/hiv-aids/medications-list.

[57] Consroe, Paul et al. "Controlled Clinical Trial of Cannabidiol In Huntington's Disease." *Pharmacology Biochemistry and Behavior* 40, no. 3 (November 1991): 701–08. doi:10.1016/0091-3057(91)90386-G.

[58] Sagredo, O. et al. "Neuroprotective Effects of Phytocannabinoid-Based Medicines in Experimental Models of Huntington's Disease." *Journal of Neuroscience Research* 89, no. 9 (September 2011): 1509–18. doi:10.1002/jnr.22682.

[59] Beadle, Alexander. "CBD Could Treat Inflammatory Bowel Disease, Says New Study." Analytical Cannabis. May 13, 2019. https://www.analyticalcannabis.com/articles/cbd-could-treat-inflammatory-bowel-disease-says-new-study-311677.

[60] Hoffenberg, Edward J. et al. "Cannabis Oil Use by Adolescents and Young Adults with Inflammatory Bowel Disease." *Journal of Pediatric Gastroenterology and Nutrition* 68, no. 3 (March 2019): 348–52. doi:10.1097/MPG.0000000000002189.

[61] WebMD. "What's the Difference Between IBS and IBD?" Accessed August 11, 2019. https://www.webmd.com/ibs/ibd-versus-ibs.

[62] Wikipedia Contributors. "Irritable Bowel Syndrome." Wikipedia. Last modified September 12, 2019. https://en.wikipedia.org/wiki/Irritable_bowel_syndrome.

[63] Russo, Ethan B. "Clinical Endocannabinoid Deficiency Reconsidered: Current Research Supports the Theory in Migraine, Fibromyalgia, Irritable Bowel, and Other Treatment-Resistant Syndromes." *Cannabis and Cannabinoid Research* 1, no. 1 (July 2016): 154–65. doi:10.1089/can.2016.0009.

[64] Hasenoehrl, C., M. Storr, and R. Schicho. "Cannabinoids for Treating Inflammatory Bowel Diseases: Where Are We and Where Do We Go?" *Expert Review of Gastroenterology & Hepatology* 11, no. 4 (April 2017): 329–37. doi:10.1080/17474 124.2017.1292851.

[65] Lupus Foundation of America. "New Study Seeks to Determine Effectiveness of Synthetic Cannabinoid in Relieving Joint Pain in Lupus." Last modified April 17, 2018. https://www.lupus.org/news/new-study-seeks-to-determine-effectiveness -of-synthetic-cannabinoid-in-relieving-joint-pain-in-lupus.

[66] Migraine Research Foundation. "Migraine Facts." Accessed August 11, 2019. https://migraineresearchfoundation.org/about-migraine/migraine-facts.

[67] Lochte, Bryson C., Alexander Beletsky, Nebiyou K. Samuel, and Igor Grant. "The Use of Cannabis for Headache Disorders." *Cannabis and Cannabinoid Research* 2, no. 1 (2017). doi:10.1089/can.2016.0033.

[68] Rhyne, Danielle N., Sara L. Anderson, Margaret Gedde, and Laura Borgelt. "Effects of Medical Marijuana on Migraine Headache Frequency in an Adult Population." *Pharmacotherapy: The Journal of Human Pharmacology and Drug Therapy* 36 (2016): 505–10. doi:10.1002/phar.1673.

[69] Rhyne et al, "Effects of Medical Marijuana."

[70] GW Pharmaceuticals. "Sativex." Accessed August 25, 2019. https://www .gwpharm.com/healthcare-professionals/sativex#.

[71] EMC. "Sativex Oromucosal Spray." Accessed August 25, 2019. https://www .medicines.org.uk/emc/product/602/.

[72] EMC. "Sativex Oromucosal Spray."

[73] Fagan, S. G., and V. A. Campbell. "The Influence of Cannabinoids on Generic Traits of Neurodegeneration." *British Journal of Pharmacology* 171 (October 2013): 1347–60. doi:10.1111/bph.12492.

[74] Laun, A. S., and Z. H. Song. "GPR3 And GPR6, Novel Molecular Targets for Cannabidiol." *Biochemical and Biophysical Research Communications* 490, no. 1 (August 2017): 17–21. doi:10.1016/j.bbrc.2017.05.165.

[75] Gurevich, T. "The Effects of Cannabis on Hypokinetic and Hyperkinetic Movement Disorders." *Clinical Neuropharmacology* 40, no. 6: 268–72.

[76] Mayo Clinic Staff. "Post-Traumatic Stress Disorder (PTSD)." Mayo Clinic. Accessed September 15, 2019. https://www.mayoclinic.org/diseases-conditions/post-traumatic-stress-disorder/symptoms-causes/syc-20355967.

[77] Bitencourt, Rafael M., and Reinaldo, N. Takahashi. "Cannabidiol as a Therapeutic Alternative for Post-Traumatic Stress Disorder: From Bench Research to Confirmation in Human Trials." *Frontiers in Neuroscience* 12 (2018): 502. doi:10.3389/fnins.2018.00502.

[78] Bitencourt and Reinaldo, "Cannabidiol as a Therapeutic Alternative."

[79] U.S. National Library of Medicine. "Cannabidiol and Prolonged Exposure." ClinicalTrials.gov. Accessed September 15, 2019. https://clinicaltrials.gov/ct2/show/NCT03518801.

[80] Hayakawa, Kazuhide, Kenichi Mishima and Michihiro Fujiwara. "Therapeutic Potential of Non-Psychotropic Cannabidiol in Ischemic Stroke." *Pharmaceuticals* 3, no. 7 (July 2010). doi:10.3390/ph3072197.

[81] Hayakawa et al, "Therapeutic Potential."

[82] Hayakawa, K. et al. "Repeated Treatment with Cannabidiol But Not Delta9-Tetrahydrocannabinol Has a Neuroprotective Effect without The Development of Tolerance." *Neuropharmacology* 52, no. 4 (March 2007): 1079–87. doi:10.3390/ph3072197.

[83] Schurman, Lesley D., and Aron H. Lichtman. "Endocannabinoids: A Promising Impact for Traumatic Brain Injury." *Frontiers in Pharmacology* 8 (2017): 69. doi:10.3390/ph3072197.

[84] Kossen, Jeremy. "Can Cannabis Prevent and Treat Traumatic Brain Injury?" Leafly. July 24, 2016. https://www.leafly.com/news/science-tech/cannabis -and-traumatic-brain-injury.

[85] Key to Cannabis. "How to Use CBD for Concussions and Traumatic Brain Injuries." Accessed August 11, 2019. https://keytocannabis.com/blogs/cannabis/how -to-use-cbd-for-concussions-and-traumatic-brain-injuries.

INDEX

R

Resing, Charlotte, 13

S

Sex, and dosages, 53
Stroke, 102–104
Suppositories, 38

T

Tetrahydrocannabinol (THC), 7, 8,
   18–19, 28–29
Tinctures, 7, 28, 33
Transdermal patches, 30, 38
Traumatic brain injury (TBI), 104–106

U

Ulcerative colitis, 85–87

V

Vape pens, 30, 34–35

W

"War on drugs," 12–14
Weight and dosages, 52–53

ABOUT THE AUTHORS

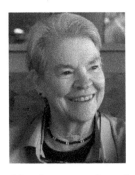

Alice O'Leary Randall is a senior spokesperson for the medical cannabis movement, cofounded in 1976 with her late husband, Robert C. Randall, the first person in the United States to legally receive medical cannabis. For more than two decades, Robert and Alice worked tirelessly to reform the prohibitions against cannabis. After Robert's death in 2001, Alice became a hospice nurse and later a grief counselor. She retired in 2012 and reentered the medical cannabis field. She frequently writes and speaks on the issue. Working with Mary's Medicinals of Denver, she developed the Cannabis Primer series in 2015 and Mary's Prime Time in 2017 (www.maryspubs.com). She has served on the board of directors for the American Cannabis Nurses Association and the advisory board for United in Compassion, an Australian medical cannabis organization. Her book *Medical Marijuana in America: Memoir of a Pioneer* was first released in April 2014. Her most recent publication is *Mary's Cannabis Primers Collection: Vol. I.* Both titles are available on Amazon. Find Alice at www.aliceolearyrandall.com.

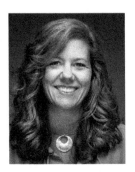

Eloise Theisen is a board-certified adult geriatric nurse practitioner with over 20 years' experience in nursing. With Dr. David Ferrera, Eloise started her own cannabis practice in 2014, treating more than 5,500 patients using cannabis. In 2018 she cofounded Radicle Health in Walnut Creek, California (www.radiclehealthcare.com). She is president-elect of the American Cannabis Nurses Association.